MW01519664

GRAY MAN

AN AVERAGE MAN'S JOURNEY TO PERSONAL GREATNESS

Brett Sobieraski

Gray Man- An Average Man's Journey to Personal Greatness

Copyright © 2022 by Brett Sobieraski

ISBN: 979-8-9863097-0-5 (paperback)

ISBN: 979-8-9863097-1-2 (eBook)

No part of this publication may be reproduced, stored in a retrieval system, or transmitted in any form or by any means, electronic, mechanical, photocopying, recording, or otherwise without written permission of the Publisher.

For information regarding permission, write to:
Brett Sobieraski
Bas813@yahoo.com

Printed in the United States of America

Editor: Sheila Kennedy, The Zebra Ink

Cover Design: Jackie Zimmerman, Queen of GSD

Interior Formatting: Word-2-Kindle

To my mother and father,
thank you for never making me feel gray
and I look forward to your visits.

Foreword

By Todd Baxter

Knowing I would be writing this for a person that defines perseverance, illustrates grit, and demonstrates overcoming intense physical fitness and mental challenge each day of his life, I felt unworthy. I needed motivation. I waited to write until after I finished an exercise routine in my basement; intervals on the bike, immediately followed by supersets to keep the cardio up for 30 minutes. Thinking of Sergeant Brett Sobieraski at the completion, gasping to breathe, tired, I recognized how good my workout actually was not, not in comparison to Brett.

We should all have that challenge, that creative tension, which motivates us. Peter Senge coined the term "creative tension" in his 1990 book, *The Fifth Discipline: The Art and Practice of the Learning Organization*, to describe the gap between where a group or person is and where they want to go — between vision and reality or desired results.

In this book, Brett illustrates top quality, beginner-friendly, long-hauled mental and physical improvement. Through this reading you will find that we all have raw primal abilities to strive harder, push limits, and drive us to new goals. Sure, blood, sweat, tears, aches, bad emotional days, and setbacks are part of any routine, but we can all move forward and keep telling ourselves, "You are doing it."

Also, if you ever wondered if having a toilet bowl full of foam after you pee is a good thing, then this book is for you.

Brett was not always a great athlete. At one time he was in poor shape, a smoker, who was disappointed by the example he was displaying to his sons. By becoming a part of an elite community, a police department's SWAT team, Brett found membership that required outstanding levels of physical fitness and mental toughness. The mission of a SWAT officer is dangerous and demands one to be highly skilled in essential tasks, to overcome every obstacle, to be a strong leader, yet at the same time to be humble in heart with a love for others.

This became Brett's driving factor, to become the very best he could be. To move from the gray area of an average person going through life, to an arena of personal greatness. This truly transformed him. Brett is not talking about someone else's prominence, but his own personal challenge and perseverance. That is key as you read and feel his transformation. This is about self-improvement and the individual accomplishment at your level. It is about becoming free of your baggage and in control of your own destiny.

This story of personal transformation really begins with the fact that Brett is just an overall good person.

Any noble accomplishment is built on the foundation of character. You will see Brett giving continuously to others. In fact, Brett was recognized with the Henry H. Jensen Memorial Award, presented annually since 1936 to an unsung hero in law enforcement. Brett's service to our community includes raising more than $80,000 for such organizations as the Veterans Outreach Center, New York State Special Olympics, Huntington Disease, and the All In All The Time Foundation.

Brett's recipe for accomplishment then builds with knowledge. One can see Brett dig into what he sets his mind to and studies the challenge like he was going into battle against it. Self-improvement is as simple or complicated as you want to make it. Next is the effort. This is up to you, but you will realize that any effort forward on a continuous basis moves you out of the gray.

Brett challenges all of us to turn our humble existence into a life that includes a focus on our best physical and mental health, increased self-confidence, greater strength, longevity, a life filled with love for self and more importantly helping others. In the pages ahead Brett takes us on that journey with him...and shows us the way. Rest assured the information you are going to gain is fully assessed and tested with blood and sweat. You will find your worth, progressively driving towards it, in a never-ending quest for a finish line, until we all meet our fate at the ultimate finish line six feet in the ground. Live it the best you can.

I leave you with a verse from the Bible which best illustrates Brett.

For this very reason, make every effort to add to your faith goodness; and to goodness, knowledge; and to knowledge, self-control; and to self-control, perseverance; and to perseverance, godliness; and to godliness, mutual affection; and to mutual affection, love.
2 Peter 1:5-7

TABLE OF CONTENTS

Introduction

A gray man is someone who moves around the periphery without creating any stimulus. He blends into his surroundings and is overlooked, unnoticed and forgotten, mostly because he is average. This perfectly described both my childhood and most of my adult life. I began as and was the consummate gray man and stood out at nothing. I was Mr. Average at most things and less than average when it came to athleticism. The world is chock full of people like me. I think of it as a bell curve with 10% being on the very low end, 10% on the very high end with the remaining 80% in the middle being various shades of gray. I was gray through and through. At times it was frustrating but eventually I had accepted it. It took me many years to learn that personal greatness is still obtainable for average folks like me. It wasn't until I looked past my lack of physical attributes and focused on my mental toughness, that I began experiencing personal successes. This is my journey.

Chapter 1- My Gray Origins

"The average man does not want to be free. He simply wants to be safe." – H L Mencken

Growing up in Lockport, NY, it was easy to feel average. It was a safe, rather gray, city situated about 30 miles east of Niagara Falls. It was, by all accounts, your average small city with a population of roughly 20,000 and the town of Lockport was the same size.

I walked to both elementary and junior high school. It wasn't until high school that I needed to ride a bus. There was a small downtown section and a much larger commercial area in the town. The community as a whole was very safe and I either walked or rode my bike wherever I went. It was only on rare occasions did my parents need to give me a ride. There were two different city parks close to my house and a small convenience store only two blocks away. I would often spend my allowance buying candy there. The standing rule was I needed to be home before the streetlights turned on. Once old enough, I had a paper route and would deliver them on the way to the YMCA where I would often play floor hockey or foosball. I graduated high school with 400 other students and knew most of them by name. Lockport was a great place to grow up, but it undoubtedly fostered my grayness. It also planted a seed for my personal greatness.

As the middle child of a family of five, there was my older sister, Julie, and little sister, Shari. I loved my sisters but always remembered wanting to have a brother to pal around with. My father, John, was a detective at the Lockport Police Department. He didn't make enough money at the time, so he worked another nearly full-time job at a local metal plating company, as well as remodeling jobs on the weekends. I remember him not being home much as a child, but he was certainly my idol. I wanted to be just like him which included the overwhelming desire to be in law enforcement. My mother, Diane, on the other hand, was a stay-at-home mom and was always around.

I viewed them differently. My father was rather stern, fearless, and hardened. He never showed much emotion. I knew he loved me, but he never said it. My mother was kind and gentle. She saw the good in everyone, and I never heard her speak ill of people. Her smile was sweet and always genuine. Mom loved to walk everywhere and always remained physically fit. She enjoyed going to the YMCA for aerobics classes and to swim.

As for me, I was a shy kid with a speech impediment that made me sound like I had an accent. My childhood physician, Dr. Muscato, was a gruff man who would ask my mother, "Where the hell did you get that kid, New York City?" At times I was difficult when it came to getting shots and he would tell her, "He's acting like a piss-pot and needs a good slap." My mother was much too kind to ever strike me.

Many of my summers were spent at a public park down the street playing basketball, softball, and ping pong. It became evident to me that I wasn't very athletic after often being picked last for impromptu games. Not being picked last was considered a big win for me. I was most certainly below average for my age when it came to God given athletic talents. I played organized baseball and soccer but sat the bench most of the time. I remember one baseball game that was especially important to the team and the coaches never put me in the game. Inning after inning, I kept anticipating going in because the rules stated each team member was required to play a minimum of two innings. To make matters worse, I was the only extra player and sat by myself on the bench while my teammates were on the field. At school I was a middle-of-the-road B average student. My entire youth was spent as the gray child, never standing out at anything, and often overlooked.

My grayness continued into junior high school. I would again get picked nearly last for our weekend football or basketball games. I wasn't good enough to make the junior varsity baseball and basketball teams and my parents forbid me to play football. I did join the track team because there were no cuts. I initially tried the long jump and triple jump but was horrible at it. The coaches steered me towards running and I liked it. I mostly competed in the one mile and two-mile events and would always finish at the back of the pack.

During this time I met Paul Haenle, who would become my best friend. He was smarter than I was or, at the bare minimum, studied much harder than I did. If necessary, he would stay up late to complete his homework while I would half-ass it and call it a night. It was my first lesson in the fact that you get out exactly what you put in. This caused me to study harder and slowly I was starting to become more of an A student as opposed to a B student.

Once in high school, among 1200 students, I stared in awe of the upperclassmen who walked the halls with their varsity letter jackets. They would have large letter "L" on both the front and back, with the sports they played embroidered on it. Most were three sport athletes and had numerous patches on the sleeves that read "Sectional Qualifier," "Sectional Champion" and "State Qualifier." An elite few sported "State Champion" patches. I looked at these people as gods and wanted a jacket in the worst way.

For track and field, one needed to accumulate a certain number of points by finishing in the top three during meets. The higher you placed the more points you would receive. By this time I had transitioned to the intermediate hurdles which was a relatively new event for high school track. It was 440 yards long with 10 evenly spaced 36" hurdles. Two-time gold medal Olympian hurdler Edwin Moses quickly became my idol.

It was during this year I met Fran McKenna. He had attended different elementary and junior high schools, so I had never met him before high school. We immediately became friends and in a relatively short amount of time Paul, Fran and I were like the Three Musketeers.

I spent my sophomore year running mostly Junior Varsity Track and had zero chance of earning a varsity letter. My junior year included many varsity races, and I could only muster one third place finish against a poorly fielded team. I was steadily maturing into a gray man. I am still disappointed when I think of what happened next.

In the early spring of my senior year I had a varicocele surgery to correct an enlarged vein in my groin area. I had fully recovered in time for the upcoming track season, but I had thrown in the towel. I lied and told the coaches my doctor said I shouldn't run for several months. I knew there was no way in hell I was going to earn my varsity letter, so I had completely given up.

After graduation I attended the Rochester Institute of Technology (RIT) for my first year of college. I liked the college experience except for the classes. I thought they were boring and began spending more time drinking beer than studying. Before long, the school year was winding down and Fran had told me he had joined the Army Reserves and would be attending boot camp that summer. I had never given the military much thought as a young adult but in my childhood, I had been obsessed with it. I remember reading a book entitled *Leathernecks* dozens of times. It told of the duties and adventures of United States Marine Corp soldiers. Fran went on to tell me that he was on a split option, meaning he would attend basic training that summer followed by advanced training the following summer. It was designed for college students. My only other option at the time was to return to the Pizza Oven in Lockport where I had worked since I was 15.

Without telling my parents, I located a recruiter in Rochester and began the process to join the New York Army National Guard. After signing on the dotted line for the Military Occupational Specialty (MOS) of 92 Bravo-Military Intelligence, I informed my parents, who were now divorced, of my intentions. My father had served in the Army and was lukewarm on the idea. My mother was rather upset and acted as if I was going off to war. I convinced her I would be fine, but she was still sad I was leaving for the summer.

When my departure day came, I wasn't sure if I was more anxious about the flight to Fort Knox, Kentucky, or the actual boot camp, because I had never been on a plane. I spent two days at the base before being informed that they did not have room for many of us and we would be going to Fort Jackson in South Carolina. Over 40 of us piled on to a Greyhound bus and, even at my young age, I was surprised when the drill sergeant walked away after the bus door closed. Uncle Sam was sending us there without any supervision. I wasn't surprised at what happened next. At the first stop, guys piled back on the bus carrying cases of beer, cartons of cigarettes and Playboy magazines. It felt like a tour bus going to a concert or football game. We paid hell upon arriving at the new Army base when the drill sergeants noticed many of my comrades were drunk.

I attended basic training for eight weeks and fell in love with it. I liked the structure, the marching, the physical training, the hardship, the camaraderie and even the food. I applied myself and would do better than most at the various learned skills. One part of me thought I was finally losing my "grayness," but I was still skeptical.

Many of my peers came from larger cities and talked about robbing people or other various run-ins with the law. They said their choices were going to prison or enlisting in the Army. Others came from very rural areas and said this was the only job they could find. I grew up somewhat sheltered and all of this surprised me, but I still felt proud of what I was accomplishing.

The only negative was the "hurry up and wait" mentality. They would put us in formation for what felt like an hour under the beating sun before the next training evolution. I'm sure some of it was by design but it happened all the time. Regardless of that, I loved it so much that I wanted to stay. Other recruits told me how they were going to infantry training after and were guaranteed airborne school. I requested and was granted a meeting with my Commanding Officer. I explained I did not want to leave after boot camp but rather enlist in the regular Army. Unfortunately, he explained to me I needed to return home for six months before doing so.

The regular Army had an agreement with the state National Guard units because in the past the Guard would lose numerous soldiers like me and a "cooling off" period hoped to alleviate that.

I returned at the end of summer lean and mean but without a plan. Continuing at RIT was not possible because of financial reasons, and now I needed to find a job. After some searching, I landed a part time job at a carpet store. I was still in army mode and would do push-ups, sit-ups and run first thing in the morning. That lasted about a month and slowly faded away the same way my desire to enlist full time in the Army did.

Fran also began working at the carpet store while still going to college and we did everything together. He would date a girl and I would date that girl's friend. We would lift weights together, eat lunch together and hit the bars together. If someone saw me without him, they would ask where he was and vice versa. We were as close as brothers and our respective parents treated us like their sons. We were both pursuing a career in law enforcement and always talked about working together one day -- how we would be a two-man wrecking crew for criminals. Rarely would a day go by without us seeing one another. He was my best friend and always there for me.

What happened next in my life still boggles my mind. I can't fully explain all of the "whys" but the main one being the influence my father had over me, and my desire to be like him. I found myself walking into Wilson

Farms Convenient Mart in downtown Lockport and buying the same brand of cigarettes he smoked. He had been a chain smoker for as long as I could remember. None of my friends were smokers and I had never tried them before but that didn't stop me from buying them. I lit one up after returning to my car and nearly coughed myself to death. That also didn't stop me, and soon after I became a regular smoker. It all happened so fast which is the case in many other types of addiction.

I returned to college at Niagara County Community College, while nearly working full time at the carpet store, and really enjoyed it. I felt I had matured since RIT and the class work was interesting. I graduated with a 3.55 grade point average and continued on to Buffalo State College. The momentum continued through the first year with straight As except for a B in a music course I was forced to take. During that time I was encouraged by my father to take the civil service test for the Lockport Police Department (LPD). I never had a strong desire to work in my hometown. I loved where I lived but I didn't want to arrest or intervene in the lives of people I knew on a first name basis. Another factor was I mistakenly believed being a police officer in Lockport would be boring, and I was looking for the opposite of that. I wanted excitement plus room for advancement. The Lockport Police Department had 50 officers and little opportunity to do anything other than patrol work. Thus, I had set my sights on working at the federal level or at the bare minimum, a large metropolitan city.

Even though I was a gray man I always had a tendency to have visions of grandeur. In my early years it was a curse because I could never live up to them like parading down the high school halls sporting a varsity letter jacket. Later in my life, this way of thinking would eventually be responsible for diving headfirst into future herculean challenges. My father rightfully explained that it was always good to have options. I scored well on the test, and, after an interview, I was offered the job. I reluctantly took it while reminding myself that I could always take another job down the road. I began my law enforcement career with the LPD on May 10th, 1988, at the ripe age of 21.

Chapter 2- Becoming Less Gray

In late summer, I began the police academy and loved it just as I did Army basic training and for all the same reasons. My time at Fort Jackson had made me tougher both physically and mentally. It had taken away a little of the gray I had felt my whole life. For the first time ever, I singularly focused on being my best. I lived and breathed the academy life. Even though I was now a smoker, I could run 1.5 miles faster than anyone in the academy, clocking in a time of nine minutes flat. I called it being "cop fast" because I was still only average in the real world. One of the directors of the academy, Captain James Gray of the Niagara Falls Police Department, was an ex-smoker and had constantly tried to get me to quit. His trick was a rubber band around his wrist. He demonstrated how he would stretch it, then snap himself whenever the urge to smoke would happen. I appreciated his efforts, but I had no intentions of quitting.

I ended up with the overall academy award for excellence at graduation. For the first time in my life I wasn't the gray man and it felt indescribably great. My father pinned my badge on my uniform during graduation and I could see pride in his hardened eyes. It was extra special because he had just recently retired, and "my" badge was the one he had worn throughout his 28-year career. My mother cried tears of joy and couldn't stop hugging me. Things came full circle for me 27 years later when I pinned my badge to my oldest son's shirt as

my father watched in the audience. It was an exceptionally proud dad moment for me.

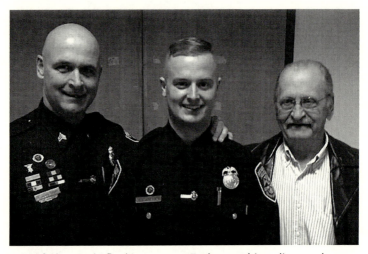

My father and I flanking my son Zachary at his police academy
graduation ceremony in 2015.

I settled in as a police officer and really enjoyed the
job and the brotherhood I shared with my fellow officers. Officers like Larry Eggert, Mike Niethe, and Scott
Seekins trained and mentored me along the way. Less
than a year after the academy graduation, I was called
into the chief's office and was told Captain Gray wanted
me to return and assist in instructing physical training.
There was a caveat though and you guessed it, I needed
to quit smoking. On the spot I handed over my pack of
cigarettes to the chief. I quit smoking for close to a week
but could no longer resist the urge. I essentially became
a closet smoker at work and still taught the physical

training. The simple truth is people can want you to stop an addiction and dangle all types of carrots in front of you, but you have to want to stop. You need your own reason to stop, and I hadn't found one.

On January 4, 1991, my fiancé Jacki gave birth to our son Zachary Andrew. He was absolutely perfect, and we had moved into my father's old house he had recently remodeled. Being a great father, he sold it to us at a bargain price.

There was an urgent knock on the door on June 8th during the middle of the night. I answered it to see a fellow police officer I had gone to high school with, Lamar Cousins. He told me Fran had been in a bad car accident and wasn't sure if Fran was alive. After working as a peace officer at a college in Buffalo, Fran became a New York State Trooper and was assigned to the Alexandria Bay area in northern NY. The summers were extremely busy due to tourism, but the winters were long and boring. We had talked several months before and were trying to figure out how we could work together. LPD did not accept transfers and we thought maybe the Buffalo Police Department might be a viable option. We agreed each of us would do some homework on the matter.

My gut told me Fran was dead because deep inside I could sense it. He had gone out to dinner with a fellow trooper who had become legally intoxicated and, on the ride home the trooper, at a very high rate of speed, flipped his car over killing Fran and injuring himself. One of Fran's brothers later confided in me that Fran had told him this trooper would often drive fast both on and off duty. The local State Police thought it was better that I inform his parents because of our close friendship. It was the hardest thing I've ever done telling them and his sister Maura that Fran had died. I am crying now as I write this. Eight of his other nine brothers and sisters began arriving at his parents' house and the story of his death had to once again be told. Each time the hole in my heart grew bigger and by the time I left, there wasn't much left of it. I remember eventually returning home and crying myself to sleep. Jacki and I were married on June 29th, and I was deeply saddened that Fran wasn't there. My youngest son, Gabriel Frances, born absolutely perfect two years later, bears his name.

I was unaware of it then, but I did not allow myself to fully grieve for Fran because it hurt so much. The brother I had always longed for was suddenly gone and it led to emotions of both anger and disbelief. Memories of him would pop into my head and I would try to think of something else because the pain was so intense. Friends would mention his name and I would quickly change the subject. Instead of working through those feelings, I buried them the same way people who suffer from Post Traumatic Stress Disorder (PTSD) do. I saw pain and unfairness every day at work and had developed a means for internalizing it, so I could maintain my sanity and a positive outlook. I couldn't do this with Fran because I was too close to the pain and suffering. I was afraid it would consume me. It took me many years to tackle this, and I have many "Brothers" to thank. Brothers I had not yet met at that time.

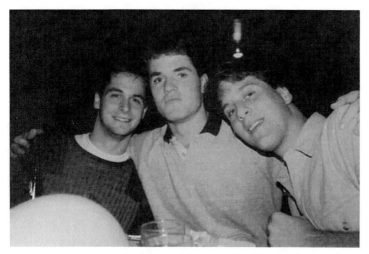

Me, Fran, and good friend Jim Hildreth circa 1986

Chapter 3- The Big Move

Later in 1991, just before Christmas, the mayor of Lockport ordered layoffs to include four police officers. I was safe because I had seniority over several other officers. These officers began searching for jobs and learned that the Rochester Police Department (RPD) accepted lateral transfers, meaning you only needed to go through a very abbreviated academy and shortened field training. Better yet, Captain Bob Wale of the RPD grew up in Lockport and his father retired as the Chief of Detectives for the LPD. He was willing to fast track the application process for me. The more I learned of the RPD, the more it piqued my interest.

Shortly after joining the LPD, I had developed a keen interest in making drug arrests. Traffic and parking tickets didn't nearly interest me as much as marijuana and cocaine arrests. Our department assigned one detective to a county-wide drug task force run by the Niagara County Sheriff's Department. I would often meet up with Detective Larry Eggert when he was assigned there to pass on narcotics information. He would tell me of his cases and undercover work. I was completely mesmerized and wanted that assignment in the worst way. The roadblock was my lack of seniority on the job and there were many officers, with more time, who also wanted it.

After discussions with Jacki and my father, I decided I would resign and transfer to the RPD with the other four officers. Although it was a bold move, I strongly believed there would be many more opportunities in a 700-person department than the 50-person department I was working in. On February 2nd, 1992, I began my career with the RPD. During my field training I was assigned to the Highland Section which was a nicer part of the city. In a way it reminded me of Lockport. I was then permanently assigned to the Clinton Section working the midnight shift. At first, I couldn't believe the amount of poverty and crime in that northeast part of the city. I had rarely ventured into Rochester while attending RIT and had always thought of it as a middle-class city because of the major companies there such as Kodak, Bausch and Lomb and AC Delco. It was definitely an eye opener coming from my hometown of Lockport that didn't have nearly close to the same amount of poverty. We eventually bought a house in the rural town of Hamlin. It was a 40-minute commute to work and only a 45-minute drive back to Lockport.

I continued to make narcotics arrests and it was a target rich environment. I wanted desperately to get assigned to the department's Special Investigation Section (SIS) where undercover narcotics officers worked.

I had two near death incidents while working as a patrol officer that were closely spaced together. In the fall of 1995, I was temporarily assigned to SIS and the section Lieutenant Bo Beam joked they needed me off road patrol before I got killed. The assignment became permanent on the first of the year. I was truly living a dream buying drugs and kicking in doors during the execution of high-risk narcotic search warrants. I grew my hair down to my shoulders and sported a goatee. I even put my earring back in that I had secretly gotten in high school from a friend who numbed my ear with ice and stuck a giant needle through it with a potato as a backstop. The job was everything I had expected and more. I couldn't believe they were paying me to go to work. I would have done it for free!

While assigned there I reluctantly took the sergeant exam. I didn't score near the top, but I wasn't disappointed because I loved my current assignment. As luck would have it, the department restructured and created more sergeant jobs. I had strongly contemplated turning down the promotion until Captain Wale, now in charge of SIS, told me he would throw me out of the unit if I did not take it. I was sad the day I had to cut my hair, shave my face, and remove the earring.

I was promoted to the rank of sergeant on July 28, 1997, with Jacki and my two sons looking on as well as my parents. I saw that same look of pride in my father's eyes, and my mother's eyes watered with tears of joy. My young boys looked up at me in amazement as I repeated the oath of office. I had mixed emotions but deep down I knew it was the right move.

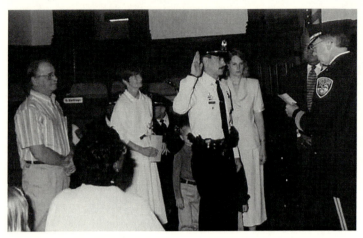

Surrounded by family at my promotion ceremony in 1997

There was an opening on the midnight shift in the Clinton Section and I was hoping to land there. The hours would be better for the family, and I considered that part of the city home. That didn't happen and I was ordered to report to the Genesee Section, on the other side of the city, to work the afternoon shift from 2:45 pm to 11:00 pm. I was disappointed both because I wasn't familiar with the section and the hours were terrible for my family life. I knew I was going to miss dinners, school functions and bedtime with my sons. What I didn't know was it would put me on a course to meet two men that proved to be very influential in my life, Pete Brunett and Aaron Springer.

Pete had just been promoted to Lieutenant and was my new direct supervisor commanding the platoon. He was a man that had the energy and enthusiasm of ten. He treated those under his command like family and was always there for them. He led from the front and gave 110% all of the time without exception. He had served for numerous years on the Special Weapons and Tactics (SWAT) Team, and tales of his service were legendary. He soon became my mentor, and I learned all my supervisory skills from him.

The platoon was made up of mostly rookie officers that had not been out of the academy for long. One of those officers was Aaron Springer, who had recently left the Army. He was young and enthusiastic with a mild chip on his shoulder. He was also a bit of a Neanderthal and at one time nearly led the department in usage of force during arrests. I saw enormous potential under the surface and did my best to mentor him. There were certainly bumps in the road like the one time he refused to take a stolen car report from a gentleman because of the questionable circumstances surrounding it. The gentleman called in a complaint, and I assured him Officer Springer would return to take the report. At this point in time Aaron had several other personnel complaints pending in Internal Affairs and didn't need another. After ordering him to take the report I could see he was agitated. At the end of the shift I asked him where the report was, and with a straight face he told me he hadn't had time to return and take it. I knew this was a lie and called him into my office because I didn't want to explode in front of his peers. I opened up our departmental General Orders which was in a five-inch binder that weighed a ton. I turned to the section on Stolen Vehicles and asked him to point out where it said the man should not get a report. He began to open his mouth to offer an excuse and before he spit it all out, I threw the book at him, striking him in the face with it. I didn't learn that from Pete, but I knew it was necessary. Aaron looked shocked and I followed up that he would leave at once to take the report and I had better not see an overtime slip from him. Before leaving he acknowledged that he was wrong and was fiercely loyal to me from there on out.

Fast forward 10 years later and Aaron had earned his Associates, Bachelors, and Masters Degrees. He went from being somewhat of a knuckle dragger, to one of the most intelligent, insightful, and effective leaders in the department. He would work his way up to become Commander of the SWAT Team and was held in the highest regard by those who served under him. Eventually he would become my boss and mentor.

In 1999, crack cocaine was the scourge of Rochester, and the associated violence was on a sharp incline. The war on drugs had kicked into full gear and SIS added two new narcotics teams. I applied and was selected to head one of them. I was happy beyond words to be back working undercover. I had a gung-ho group of six officers, and we rained hell upon the drug dealers in the Genesee and Downtown Sections of the city. I was back in my element and never took another promotional exam. It was a miracle I had returned to SIS so quickly and, I knew beyond a shadow of a doubt, it would not happen if I became a lieutenant.

Chapter 4- Time for a Change

It was a night just like any other in 2001, as my family sat around in the kitchen playing a game after dinner. There was a tub of pretzel rods on the table, and we were enjoying them as a snack while playing Farkle. I glanced out of the corner of my eye and saw my son Gabriel pretending to smoke a pretzel rod as if it was a cigarette. My immediate instincts told me to scold him, but I quickly realized I would have been a hypocrite. After all he was just trying to be like me, much the same way I wanted to be like my father when I started smoking. A profound sense of failure came over me when I realized I had been such a poor role model. It was so heavy I wanted to cry, and I knew I needed to make a change. At that exact moment and without hesitation, I vowed to never smoke again.

I had tried to quit several times in the past but this time it was entirely different. This time it involved the safety and well-being of my child. When I awoke the next morning, I fought the extraordinarily strong urge to smoke the cigarettes I had left. After crumpling them up and throwing them in the garbage, I headed off to work. I left early enough so that I could stop at Wegmans to buy the nicotine patch which I placed on my upper back in the parking lot. As I reached a familiar stoplight, I instinctively reached to my breast pocket to grab a cigarette, it was completely involuntary. The same thing happened as I pulled into work realizing that I would always smoke a cigarette prior to entering the building. I was smart enough to know I needed to change certain habits and rituals. I began driving a different route to work and parking in a different spot upon arriving there. I even used a different door to enter the building. I temporarily gave up drinking coffee because that was a huge trigger for my smoking. It was also difficult to resist the urge to smoke after meals.

The first week was certainly the toughest but the nicotine patch really helped curb my cravings. I also knew that failure was never an option. Every time the urge to smoke would come, I would quickly think of my son Gabriel holding that pretzel rod like it was a cigarette. That in and of itself was enough to quell my craving to smoke.

After six weeks of wearing the nicotine patch, I was greatly concerned how the first day without it would be. To my surprise, I had changed enough of my routines that it was a fairly easy day to get through. I knew what the triggers were and did my best to avoid them or at the very least see them coming. While a part of me still missed smoking, a different part did not miss standing out in subzero weather or during a driving rainstorm to smoke a cigarette. It wasn't until that point that I had realized my cigarette addiction was no different than any other drug addiction. It had ruled my life while doing it and now I began to feel free.

I had been working in an offsite building where most of the people did not realize we were undercover narcotics officers. In 2002, my unit was made to move into the newly built Public Safety Building and, while roaming the hallways, I discovered they had installed a gym. It had been many, many years since I had last lifted weights or ran, but somehow, I knew this gym could help me in my battle to remain smoke-free. I went home that night and scrounged up what little gym clothes I had before realizing I did not even own a pair of sneakers that weren't grass stained from mowing the lawn. I frantically searched my closet and found the wrestling shoes I would wear while helping to coach my kid's youth wrestling team. They would have to do for the time being.

I went to bed with a huge smile on my face thinking of the glory days when I would beat most police recruits during the 1.5 mile run or the times I would lift weights with my best friend Fran. I was certain I would put a hurting on the gym the following day. Back to the glory days! Or so I thought.

It was written in the contract that personnel working in the Public Safety Building receive a one-hour lunch break. I quickly changed into my gym clothes at noon then walked into the brand-new gym, eager to get started. The first thing to catch my eye was an empty bench and I confidently placed 45-pound plates on either side of the Olympic barbell. It's the weight I would warm up with Fran back in the day. I slid onto the bench, unracked the weight and lowered it to my chest. I was surprised at how heavy it felt when I began to push the bar back up and it only moved an inch before settling back on my chest. My initial thought was, "Oh shit! I'm stuck!" I frantically looked around the room, but I was the only person in there. I tried again to lift the bar but this time it didn't even budge off my chest and panic began to set in. I lifted the bar with my left arm while lowering my right arm until the right plate slid off. This caused a violent chain reaction resulting in the left plate to then fall and crash to the floor also. It was almost like a horrific teeter totter.

I had just finished quickly stowing the plates in the rack when a civilian lady opened the gym door and asked if I was OK. Using my best acting skills I responded, "Yes," and quickly followed up with, "Why?" She said she heard two loud crashes and thought someone had gotten hurt. The building was brand new and there were loud banging noises that would happen all throughout the day. We were told it was "banging bolt syndrome" meaning the building was still settling. I replied I heard the banging too and it must've been the banging bolts. She nodded in agreement then left.

I slid 25-pound plates on the bar, thinking it might be better to start at that weight. I struggled through to get eight repetitions and wondered when I had become so weak. I did a few more sets of bench presses, followed by some overhead dumbbell presses for my shoulders, and then glanced at the line of three treadmills. One would think that the setback I just had on the bench press would have shaken me back to reality, but the glory days always seem to have a strong hold on me.

I thought back to the police academy when I would run 1.5 miles in nine minutes equating to a six-minute mile pace. I then did the math and realized I needed to set the treadmill at 10 mph.

I was fairly certain this was my first time on a treadmill, but it looked easy enough to operate. There were even preset buttons for speed. Decked out in my wrestling shoes, I climbed aboard and confidently pressed the 10 button. The belt began moving and the motor slowly began firing up like a jet engine. Before I knew it, I found myself sprinting but still moving to the rear of the machine because I could not keep up. I felt my heels at the very end of the belt and another bout of panic set in. Before I knew it, I was spit off the back of the belt but not before landing my upper body on it. I tumbled across the floor and came to rest in a heap on the other side of the gym floor. I struggled to my feet and turned the treadmill off just in time for the same lady to enter the gym again. Before she said a word I pointed to the corner of the gym and said, "The banging came from there this time." She shook her head and replied, "I sure hope this building settles soon." while walking out the door.

I wanted to leave but told myself that morning I would run 1.5 miles today. I once again stood on the treadmill but thought cutting the pace in half to 5 mph or a 12-minute mile pace might be a wiser idea. I hit the "5" button and began running. Time seemingly stood still as seconds felt like minutes and I was wheezing as if I was breathing through a straw. I began feeling dizzy and my vision started to narrow but I continued to put one foot in front of the other. Just as the distance reached one mile, I felt I could no longer continue. I quickly hit the "Stop" button and impatiently waited for the belt to stop moving. I could barely catch my breath and began coughing violently while bent over with my hands on my knees. My buddy Andy came through the door and quickly told me that I didn't look good. In between coughing jags, I told him I had a tickle in my throat, but I knew I looked like death warmed over.

After returning to my locker room changing into my work clothes, I looked into the full length mirror. I saw a dejected man and thought, *You fucking did this, so now you need to fucking undo this*. It hit me that the climb out of my self-induced pit of unhealthiness would be a difficult one.

The next morning my legs throbbed when my feet hit the floor and I wasn't sure if I would make it into the bathroom. Once in the shower I realized it was a struggle to wash my face because my chest was so sore and tight. I had to tuck my chin in order to complete the process. It was a mental struggle to gather gym clothes for the day's workout and I kept thinking, *Just be a little better than yesterday.*

Those first few months were an epic battle, and I was sore and stiff most of the time. It had become my new reality and one I could not and was not fully able to embrace at first. As a reward I bought myself off the shelf running shoes. I picked them because of the price and how they looked as opposed to how they fit but let's face it, anything was better than my wrestling shoes.

I had been running, really it was more like jogging, for a couple of months when I learned of a 5K road race at a church in nearby Greece, NY. I thought it would be great to take my boys and show off my newfound lifestyle. At this time Zachary and Gabriel were eleven and nine, respectively. I signed us all up and we excitedly drove to the church. After pinning their race bibs on, I told them to try hard and I would be waiting for them at the finish line. We meshed into the crowd of runners, and I nervously waited for the start.

The gun was fired and away we went. Both of my sons sprinted ahead of me, and I was certain I would end up passing them. After the first mile they were nowhere in sight, and I began to develop a very uncomfortable rash on the inside of my left thigh. I was running in a pair of regular boxer brief underwear under a pair of gym shorts. The underwear began bunching up causing the rash. I made it to mile two and there was still no sight of my sons. By this time I was exhausted, nearly hyperventilating and my rash had turned bloody. I kept telling myself not to stop and the rash kept getting worse.

At about a half mile from the finish line I spied Gabriel walking about 100 yards ahead of me. When I reached him and, while gasping for air, I told him to run with me. Make no mistake, I did not slow down for him. I began slowing because I was tired as hell. He obliged and when he saw the finish line in the distance, he sprinted ahead of me. I tried to keep up with him, but I just couldn't. He beat me by 20 seconds and as I crossed the finish line, I saw Zachary cheering me on.

I sincerely congratulated both of them on their efforts but inside I felt like a worthless piece of shit. Neither of my boys trained for the race and they both beat me. Yes, my two preteen sons whooped my ass and I had been the one training. As painful as my bloody rash was, it wasn't close to the pain I felt for being a failure. A failure as a father figure and a role model. I hated myself and what I had let myself become.

I had come to the fork in the road. Give up and remain this shell of a man or get fucking hard and set the example. I begrudgingly confessed to myself that I lacked mental toughness, and I was going through the motions in the gym rather than meaningful training. It was the first step in allowing myself to really change. The boys playfully busted my balls on the way home about beating me and I knew the loser never gets to dictate how the victors celebrate. I was happy for them because they were proud of their accomplishment, unlike me. It was during that ride home I vowed they would never beat me again because of my own failings. This was not because of ego, it was because I wanted to be a good father, a good teacher, and an inspiration to them. I wanted them to be better than me, but I wanted them to earn it. Today I handed it to them because of my self-imposed shortcomings. Never again would this happen but I just wasn't sure how to accomplish it.

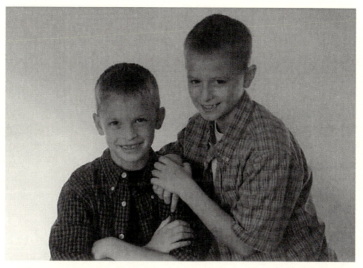

My sons Gabriel and Zachary who left me in the dust at the 5K

Chapter 5- Hard Men

On Monday, March 28, 2005, I found the answer to becoming mentally tougher although I did not initially realize it. This was the first day of a week-long SWAT school. I was attempting to become a member of my departmental SWAT Team at 38 years of age. I always had an interest in getting on the Team however when tryouts were offered the first time, after transferring to the Rochester Police Department, I did not meet the minimum amount of time to apply. The next time tryouts were offered I was working as an officer in narcotics and the unit captain did not allow us to join specialized teams. For the following tryouts I had become a uniformed platoon sergeant and they were only taking officers. Due to waning interests in joining SWAT, in 2005 they allowed both officers and sergeants to try out for the Team. I finally had my chance!

Our SWAT Team was considered a part-time unit, meaning you would work your regular duty shift day in and day out. The Team would train several days a month and occasionally for an entire week. We would be called out as needed to execute narcotics search warrants, barricaded gunmen, and other high-risk missions.

I had heard horror stories about the week-long tryout process which was led by the infamous Lieutenant Todd Baxter. I braced for the worst knowing this would not be easy. I was surprised when the first day ended and it did not seem exceedingly difficult. I did have enough common sense to realize this was the calm before the storm. Each subsequent day was harder than the last and none of them were a standard eight-hour training day. The last day included a large, barricaded gunman scenario followed by mandatory pass/fail firearm qualifications and a PT test.

We were constantly evaluated and graded throughout every minute of the week and the last part of the process was having our pictures shown on a large screen. The entire Team would then openly discuss the candidate's positives and negatives. This did not just include the past week but also interactions during regular work hours. If one person voted no, then the candidate would not be allowed on the Team. The entire class and I sat nervously down the hallway awaiting our fate. Most of us were called into the room and I remember being supremely proud that I had made the Team. Unfortunately, this was not the case for everyone in my class. Of those that did make it, we had developed an extraordinarily strong bond.

I loved SWAT training days. They reminded me of my time in the police academy and Army boot camp but on steroids. Todd squeezed out every minute out of the day and training often ran over. I remember one such day when we were all cleaning our weapons at the end of an especially hard training day and Todd was pushing us to finish. I thought it was because we were already past the allotted eight hours for the day. To my surprise, I heard Todd quietly tell someone that he had to go home and run 18 miles because he was training for a marathon. I thought that was the craziest thing I had ever heard in my life. My ass was really dragging after that training day and all I envisioned myself doing was going home to have a hot meal, prop some toothpicks in my eyes to keep them open so I could play with the kids before going to bed early. I could not comprehend someone having to run 18 miles that night.

Todd was seen as a fitness god. He had taken over the physical training in the police academy from a civilian who had run it for years. He quickly made the training more like Army boot camp physical training sessions and would never tire during training evolutions. Officers still talk about their academy days with him and how tough they were. He was as squared away as they come, very inspirational and at times more machine than man.

It was hard men like him, Aaron Springer, Fabian Rivera, Garth Mitchell, Herb McClellan, Michael Diehl, and Scott Peters that began to rub off on me. I started to understand the saying that "iron sharpens iron" and these men were as tough as nails. I tried hard to emulate them and after each training day or SWAT mission I felt myself becoming bolder and, more importantly, tougher.

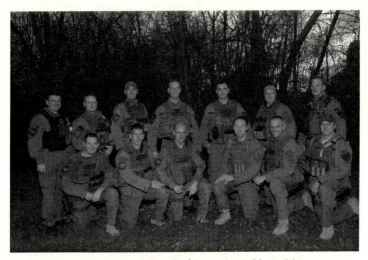

1st Row- Herb McCllellan (2nd from the left), Todd Baxter (5th from the left)

2nd Row- Mike Diehl (2nd from the left), Aaron Springer (3rd from the left)

In the fall of 2005, one of the assistant commanders of the SWAT Team approached me during a quick lunch break and was flanked by two men who sported shoulder length hair and long beards. I think he assumed I knew who they were because he only introduced them by name, Tommy Valentine and a man called Wemo. The assistant commander wanted me to work with Tommy on developing a high-risk vehicle takedown training scenario. The entire time I was wondering who the hell were these guys and my instincts told me they were special. I have always had a sixth sense for quickly sizing up people and it had kicked in. I could tell they were hardened men and were serious about what they did but I just wasn't sure who they worked for. Tommy and I agreed we would meet up the next day to plan the scenario and they left the room. I quickly found another SWAT cop and asked who the long-haired bearded guys were. I was told they were SEAL Team 6 operators. *Holy shit,* I thought, *it all made sense now.*

The correct term for their team was DEVGRU- Naval Special Warfare Development Group. SEAL Team 6 was their old name, and they are still commonly referred to as such. They are a Tier 1 unit and considered to be among the best in the world. They were in town for a week of Realistic Urban Training (RUT) and would mostly be in the Rochester area. During that week Todd had developed a friendship with Wemo and our Team helped secure residential and commercial training locations for them consisting of mostly vacant properties. We would observe their training and often do our own training nearby. I soon learned that their tactics were quite a bit different than ours. Theirs were evolving from the two wars that were raging overseas, while we were using more traditional and dated Los Angeles SWAT Team tactics. They had invented the SWAT team concept and coincidentally my Team was the second oldest in the country.

In the evenings we would take the SEALs to various Rochester restaurants and bars. Most of the time I found myself talking to Wemo and Tommy and tried my hardest not to ask too many questions. I was amazed at how smart they were, and they seemed to know everything about everything. The other trait that stuck out was their humility. I never once heard them brag or boast. Coincidentally, one of our Team's ethos was to be confident in one's ability but subdued in interactions with others. Often SWAT cops are despised for being arrogant but that was not Todd's way. Although he knew we were all alpha males, he demanded we be humble. Being a large mouth bragger was the quickest way to get booted from the Team.

Wemo, who had setup and directed the training, had greatly appreciated everything we had done for him during that time. So much so, that he had invited our team down to his Navy base in Virginia for a week to utilize their state-of-the-art training facility. Wemo had also befriended our chief of police at the time, Cedric Alexander, so it was an easy sell. Half the Team went down on March 6, 2006, and the other half the following week. We did this so that the city wasn't without our services for an entire week. We were one of only 10 SWAT Teams ever invited to their base.

It was a week I will never forget. Certain policies restricted Wemo and Tommy from actually training us and they were more like tour guides. Most days started with some type of physical training followed by shooting at one of their many ranges. We also completed training in our entry tactics at various structures. We even got to run through their obstacle course which was insanely difficult. One morning we ran a mile or so to their indoor pool. Wemo suggested a good goal would be for us to stay active in the water for 30 minutes. He further explained it could be swimming, treading water or even water walking for the non-swimmers, but the goal was to keep moving.

I had been on my local YMCA swim team as a youth but as a gray man, well actually, a gray child. I never placed in the top three at swim meets and was a less than average swimmer. I did learn to do the front crawl or freestyle stroke and the breaststroke, but I hadn't seriously swum since that time. It's hard not to be bold around men like Wemo and Tommy, so I got into an empty pool lane and began to swim free-style. Halfway down the pool I not only felt winded but also very clumsy. I made myself not stop until I reached the other end. I urgently grabbed the side of the pool upon reaching it and took in a few gulps of air to match the gulps of water I had inadvertently drank. Pushing off the wall, I began doing the breaststroke which acted as somewhat of a recovery stroke for me. Before I knew it, I had done 12 lengths of the pool and had settled into a rhythm alternating between the two swim strokes. I had always loved being in the water and with each lap I felt more comfortable. It helped that I slowed down my stroke rate and began gliding through the water as opposed to fighting it. As comfortable as it was, it seemed like time had stood still and I was feeling fatigued. I would occasionally glance up at a clock on the wall and swear it hadn't moved since the last time I had looked at it. Eventually Wemo signaled for us to stop, and I was sure I had swum much longer than 30 minutes. Much to my surprise it had only been 25 minutes, but I still felt happy I had swum the entire time.

Next, Tommy demonstrated the new pool obstacle course that he had personally developed. It was unbelievably hard and impossible for any of us to complete. Tommy did it and barely broke a sweat. I still fondly remember falling 12 feet onto my back after my grip gave out on a series of gymnastic rings.

The time our Team spent down in Virginia left an indelible mark on most of us. Once back in Rochester we began to train differently and with a different mindset. It was not all smooth sailing because some wanted to stick with the old ways but many of us fought hard to change. Wemo and Tommy had become like brothers to us and were critically important to our Team's evolution. On a personal level, those two men had become my role models and I wanted to be like them. During one conversation Wemo told me he had run a marathon and I was surprised because of his stature. He was barrel-chested and thick, but I also knew he could do whatever he put his mind to. The other surprising fact was he ran it very fast. Something about that conversation rattled around and stuck in my brain. A month later I decided to train for a half marathon race that was in September. I had studied numerous training articles and wrote down a detailed running program. This was where my mad scientist training mindset started.

At the same time I unwisely decided to take on the herculean task of building my own house. A year earlier we had bought 57 acres in nearby Carlton, New York, with the intention of putting a house on it. When I say building my own house, I do not mean being the general contractor. I did the framing, windows/doors, siding, electrical, plumbing, flooring and all the finish work. I did subcontract out the excavation, foundation, heating, insulation, and drywall work.

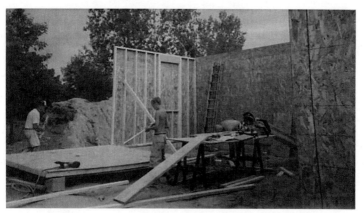

My father, son Gabriel and I working on the house

On weekdays I would wake early and get my training runs in before the sun came up. This was followed by going to work for eight hours and then immediately driving to the construction site. I would work until dark before returning home to grab a quick dinner while trying to spend a few minutes with the family. On the weekends I would work at the house from sunup to sundown. I did this all through the spring and summer and was constantly tired, but this was my new reality. My father, who knew much more about construction than I did, would come and help five or six days a week and good friends, Rich Williams, and Wayne Burchfield, would often show up to help me. Other good friends and even my young boys would pitch in on the weekends. Because of exhaustion, I would only lift weights once or twice a week and mainly for my upper body. By the end of summer my run training also began to trail off because of fatigue.

In late August, our SWAT Team was asked to assist in the search for Ralph "Bucky" Phillips in the Southern Tier area of NY. He had escaped from the Erie County Jail in April. He was almost captured several times but had a knack for getting away. During one of the instances he shot and wounded a New York State Trooper. In a second incident he ambushed two New York State Troopers that were staking out a family home. He shot both of them and one died several days later. He had turned into public enemy number one and made the FBI's 10 Most Wanted Fugitives list.

The first RPD SWAT contingent left for the Fredonia, NY command post with Todd in charge and spent a week trying to apprehend him. I led the second wave that relieved Todd and his crew. He had shown us various locations that Phillips would frequent. I remember searching vacant houses and patrolling through woods looking for him. Prior to this, I had been on well over 2000 dynamic search warrant executions while in my narcotics capacity, but this felt different. This seemed much more real, and we were fairly certain that he would not give up peacefully.

After showing us the ropes for most of the day Todd and his team departed for Rochester. I called my team of five officers together and instructed Aaron to go buy the beer and I would get the pizza. Chris Picha, a hardworking, straight as an arrow SWAT cop, gave me a perplexed look and said he thought this was a "dry" mission meaning no alcohol. Feeling my oats, I snapped back at him and told him I would determine what the mission would be.

Before getting the beer, I told Aaron I needed a favor. He drove my car from the hotel, and I would have him pull over every mile and I would spray paint a 1 then 2 and so forth on the pavement until we reached five miles. I explained to him that I wanted to run 10 miles the next morning and my training heavily involved negative splits. This meant I would try to go faster each mile and I didn't have a GPS watch at the time. This run would determine whether I would compete in the upcoming half marathon.

An hour later we all met up in a hotel room and began partaking in the pizza and beer. I would occasionally glance at Chris and see him take little baby sips from what must have been a warm beer by now. Just to piss him off I would pretend to guzzle a beer from an empty can then slam it on the dresser. I also began collecting the empty beer cans and building a pyramid by stacking them on top of each other. I would catch Aaron smirking at me because he knew how funny this was. Eventually everyone headed to their respective rooms to get some sleep, it was only 9 o'clock at night.

I was in the middle of a deep sleep when my pager began to blow up at 3 am. I called the number and was told Phillips had been stopped in a stolen car near the Pennsylvania border and fled into the woods. They needed us to get there quickly to assist in apprehending him. I rapidly assembled my Team and we headed south but not before Chris gave me the "I told you so" look. Our Team had just acquired a Bearcat, basically a 17,000 pound armored personnel carrier. Chris was heavily involved in the purchase of it and knew the vehicle front to back. I told him he was driving. He activated the emergency sirens and lights, and I will never forget the sound of the 440 hp turbo diesel spooling up. We were going down the road well over 80 mph in this giant steel can. I was riding in the back and looked across the bench seat to Aaron and we both had the "What the fuck" look as Chris began passing cars and even giant 18 wheelers on narrow country roads. At the same time we instinctively donned our armored helmets knowing we would bounce around inside that steel coffin like a pinball should we crash.

It was a white-knuckle ride for about an hour until we reached our destination. I had the eerie feeling we had crossed into Pennsylvania but now was no time to question jurisdiction. I contacted the incident commander and he told us we needed to help shore up a perimeter in the wood line on an adjacent country road. We fanned out into the triple canopy and tried to stay within eyesight of one another. More and more officers from New York and Pennsylvania began arriving and I would brief them where to go because the perimeter was still porous. Eventually most of my SWAT Team from Rochester had arrived and slowly the perimeter became airtight. I was then informed that I needed to get the full names and dates of birth of all our SWAT members because a US Marshall needed to temporarily deputize us because we were indeed in Pennsylvania.

A helicopter was hovering a short way away and we knew we were close to Phillips, but it was getting late in the day and soon it would be nightfall. Darkness would have seriously complicated the search effort and I started feeling a little helpless although we knew the perimeter needed to be maintained. There was talk that he had shot at a K9 officer earlier in the search. I really wanted to take a team to probe deeper into the forest but that was not our mission. As the sun began to set, it came across the radio that Phillips had given up and was taken into custody. At that same time you could hear a cheer starting miles away and slowly working towards us like the wave at a football stadium. We later learned that he exited the woods wearing only his underwear fearing he would be shot and killed on site.

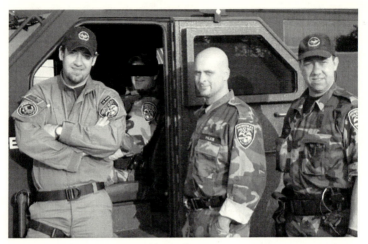

Aaron Springer, me, and Chris Picha in front of our Bearcat
in Fredonia

We piled into the Bearcat and began the trip back
to Fredonia. The small towns we passed through were
flooded with people who were cheering for us because
they knew the cop killer had been caught. Even though
our role was extremely small I was still immensely proud
to be a part of getting justice for the murdered trooper
and the two others that were shot and wounded.

We were invited to a local bar by the New York
State Police Commander who ran the operation. After a
quick shower, a handful of us jumped into a car and you
could guess who our designated driver was... Chris. The
bar was maxed out to capacity with officers celebrating
the capture. While there was a great sense of accomplishment and joy in the air, there was also a somber
undertone because a trooper had died.

The bar stayed open later than usual and it was a little after 4 am when I finally returned to the hotel. We had all agreed to meet in the hotel lobby at 9 am for the return trip back to Rochester. I was still determined to do my 10-mile run and set the alarm for 6:30 am. When it eventually went off, I fought the urge to hit the snooze button. When my feet hit the floor, I felt like crap, but I was also still riding the high that Phillips had been captured. After getting dressed, I strapped on my running shoes and headed out the door. The first mile was a little rough but then I settled into a groove, running each mile faster than the last. I was trying to take in the new views but every minute or so my mind would return to Trooper Longobardo, who was murdered by Phillips. I felt extremely sad for him and his family but used it as fuel to keep going faster. I had completed the 10 miles in less than 80 minutes and averaged around a 7:57 minute mile pace. I hadn't expected to go that fast because my run training had tapered off, but I think the added rest did me well, as did the thought of Trooper Longobardo.

After a quick shower, I headed to the continental breakfast already feeling somewhat stiff and sore from my run. Todd told me he saw me out running and I excitedly told him about the length and time of my run. Upon hearing him say it was a very solid run, I felt supremely proud. I hadn't told him or anyone else at work I was training for the half marathon. The race was only eight days away and this run did much to boost my confidence for it.

The following week flew by and before I knew it, I was among 1000 other runners jockeying for a starting position in downtown Rochester. I had arrived very early and was nervously pacing around when I noticed Todd in the crowd. Much to my surprise he was also in the race, and I think he was as equally surprised to see me. We gave each other a giant SWAT hug and he moved closer to the start of the race.

When the race finally started it was mass chaos trying to find room to run. I immediately regretted not following Todd to the front of the starting line. I tried awfully hard to run conservatively those first several miles. I fought the natural instinct of wanting to run faster to pass those that looked like they should not be ahead of me. Todd was nowhere in sight. I stuck with my game plan of running each mile faster than the last. For much of the race there was a large contingency of spectators cheering us on and it was something I had not witnessed before. I tried to thank many of the well-wishers.

I had made it through the hilly Mt. Hope Cemetery and was coming out onto Elmwood Avenue near Strong Memorial Hospital when the cheering almost became deafening. There were at least 100 spectators at the cemetery entrance/exit. I knew at this point I had a 5K or 3.1 miles remaining in the race. I was running on a path that parallels the Genesee River and was still feeling relatively strong. I suddenly noticed that Todd was about 100 yards ahead of me and I was surprised to see him. After a few minutes I was alongside him and gave him a hearty slap on the back while saying, "SWAT Tough!" He looked a little startled at first and then gave me a giant smile while telling me I was a beast. No other words were exchanged as I passed, probably because I was still in shock that I was beating the great Todd Baxter. There was 1.5 miles left in the race and I tried my best to drop the hammer and go all out. I was running fast but not as fast as I thought I should be. My body was just not cooperating with what I felt should be the plan. I was never so happy to see Frontier Field, a baseball stadium which was the finishing point. I just needed to enter the stadium and run around the warning track to the finish line. I felt as if I was finishing an Olympic marathon when I hit the warning track and the announcer said my name over the loudspeaker. I felt a big grin come across my face as I sprinted the last 100 yards.

I had finished in 1 hour 45 minutes and 36 seconds. Completely exhausted as I went to hug my wife and sons, I also felt immense pride. I felt like I was starting to become a better role model for my sons. I committed to a goal and achieved it through hard work and dedication, while still acknowledging I had faltered in training. In the midst of all these feelings, I heard the announcer say Todd's name and quickly headed towards the finish line to cheer him on. After he crossed, we again hugged, and he congratulated me. It then really sunk in that I had beat the man, the myth, the legend. Even my wife was surprised because she knew what an icon Todd was.

After about 10 minutes everything below my waist was hurting to include my feet, calves, knees, and hips but it was that good kind of pain. The pain that is earned through adversity. I eventually got into the passenger side of my wife's car and the boys were in the backseat when an excruciating feeling took over my right shoulder. I tried to ignore it at first but then it became nearly unbearable. I found myself clutching that shoulder with my left hand while rocking back and forth in the seat hoping it would make it stop. Everyone in the car knew I was in distress, and I did my best to pass it off saying I think I had a cramp in my shoulder. My wife quickly replied that she had never heard of such a thing, and I shot her a stare as if to stop talking so the boys would not get upset. It was probably the longest 40-minute car ride of my life but eventually the shoulder pain dulled as we pulled into the driveway. The next dilemma was getting out of the car because my lower body had basically seized up. It took a good one or two minutes to swing my legs out and hobble up the porch stairs to reach the inside of my house. I constantly reminded myself to remain upbeat and smile so that my boys would not see this as a "bad" thing.

Truth be told, I was sore for the following three weeks after the race and didn't run at all. I knew I needed to be better at recovering but wasn't sure how to do that. I had seen Todd during that time frame, and he looked fine. I had also seen several other of my SWAT brothers who brought up the "SWAT Tough" saying and me passing Todd on the river path. He had told them the story saying he was both impressed and proud of my effort. I thought that really spoke to his character and the type of man he was.

I went back to working on the new house, but I was feeling exceptionally burned out. It seemed like the work had slowed to a snail's pace and I began feeling like I was over my head. To make matters worse, three weeks after the race I found myself driving out to Aspen, Colorado for a five-day rifle elk hunt. I had planned the hunt before committing to building the house. It probably wasn't the best timing, but I also thought the break was just what I needed. It was a great week with many fond memories even though the paid guides were horrendous. My newfound fitness level came in handy, and I felt strong while climbing a mountain to 14,000 feet of elevation

The day after returning home from Colorado I made the 10-mile drive to the new house. I had hoped the hunting trip had recharged my batteries but that was not the case. I stood at the back of the mostly framed house and thought of all the work that needed to be done. I felt both overwhelmed and helpless and remember wishing I had never started this project which had now become the bane of my existence. Deep inside I also wished it would burn to the ground so I could get out of this mess. Looking back now, I realize I was still lacking in the mental toughness department. My intention was to put in a day's work, however, I was feeling so downtrodden, I never strapped on my tool belt, and returned home after an hour.

I had barely touched the house over the next five days and apparently my father took notice. He called me one evening and rather sternly told me we needed to get working on the house. My initial thought was to tell him he just didn't understand however, deep down I knew he did. He himself had built his own house after retiring from the Lockport Police Department. I sat quietly while he told me he knew it was going to be a long process but he was also confident we could complete it. It's funny what one phone call from a person you look up to can do. After hanging up I ordered myself to stop feeling sorry for myself. That I got myself into this and I needed to get myself out of it. Everything changed after that phone call, and I think above all I wanted to make my father proud. I started putting in extra-long days with my father next to me for most of them. He was 60 years old at the time, but you would never tell by his work ethic; the man rarely looked tired.

The house was soon sided, electrical wires were pulled through the walls, water and waste lines were fitted together and the interior was framed. It soon began to look like a house. Don't get me wrong, there were setbacks like running my waterline a quarter-mile down the road since the water main ended there. My biggest fear doing it myself was that there would be a leak and of course there was. I eventually found it and a disaster was diverted.

My dad and I, along with Rich and Wayne, worked all through the winter and into the spring. I would have never finished the house without their help. Another person that would help was my SWAT brother Herb Mc-Clellan. He didn't live far from me, and we would car-pool on SWAT training days. He is one of the most fit people I had ever met and looks like he walked out of an Under Armour catalog. He was very well respected on the SWAT Team and a man of few words. I jokingly blamed him for what happened next in my quest to find a new athletic endeavor.

My wife and I were over at his house one night when he had talked about buying a bike to do one of those "Ironman races." He said he would still ride the bike, however, gave up the thought of doing triathlons due to the swimming part of it. I was immediately intrigued about these Ironman races and peppered him with questions. He didn't have all the answers and couldn't recall the distances involved except that they were "really long." I remembered occasionally watching what I later learned were the Ironman World Championships on the television. Even though I knew very little about them, the thought of doing one rattled around and stuck in the back of my brain.

Chapter 6- Down the Rabbit Hole

In the early spring of 2007, I had completed the construction of my new home after nine long months. My building loan expired at that time, and I worked frantically over the last 60 days to pass the bank inspection. There were still a few odds and ends to do but my family was excited to move in. People who hear of the various races I have completed often ask the generic question, "What's the hardest thing you have ever done?" To this day the response has always been the same, "Building my own house," and it's never the retort they expected. I still live in that home and it's my most prized physical possession. My soul is in the walls, floors, and ceilings. Its mere presence makes me happy, and I still find myself staring at it in wonder. It was my first experience realizing that great and special things come from sacrifice, dedication, and perseverance. I loved that feeling and wanted more of it but wasn't quite sure what the next challenge would be. It didn't take long for it to reveal itself.

While packing up things in my old garage, I came across my Schwinn Premis bicycle I had purchased in 1988. It was a heavy steel framed 12 Speed road bike with the shifters on the down tube as opposed to the handlebars. I had always called it the rainbow warrior because of its colorful paint scheme. I don't think I had ridden it since 1991.

The bike jostled something loose in my brain, the thought of doing an Ironman triathlon that Herb had mentioned. This also caused me to think back to my swim in Virginia and it was like a perfect storm. That day I declared to myself that I would become an Ironman in 2007. I figured I would have the time to properly train for it since I no longer had my house construction looming over me.

This immediately caused me to do research on the Internet for a training plan. Much to my dismay this was when I first learned the official distances involved in an Ironman race-- 2.4-mile swim, 112 mile bike, followed by the 26.2 marathon. I had also learned that there were different distances in triathlons to include the Sprint, Olympic, Half Ironman and Full Ironman. I read as much as I could about triathlon training and there was a common theme from the "experts." It was that you should not attempt an Ironman in your first year of triathlon racing but rather build up to it over several years. I wondered why this was such a rule and if it was because the experts didn't, couldn't, wouldn't do one, that meant everyone else shouldn't. An officer at RPD named Kevin Chartrand was an accomplished triathlete and had competed in at least one Ironman. He pretty much gave me the same advice. He was particularly good at the sport however, I did not heed his nor the experts' advice. I bought the book *Triathlon Training Basics* by Gail Bernhardt and read it several times front to back. It became my go-to reference.

I eventually found a six-month training program on the internet that consisted of nine workouts per week. Each discipline, the swim, bike and run, would be trained three times a week. The first week initially appeared manageable and the workouts would gradually get longer over the six months. The training in months five and six looked horrifically long.

Next, I needed to find a race and was surprised that the "true" Ironman races sponsored by Ford at the time were completely sold out for the year. The sport was booming at this time, and I scoured the internet for off brand Ironman length races. I eventually found the Chesapeakeman Ultra Distant Triathlon in Cambridge, Maryland, and they were still accepting applicants for the race in September. I now had my race picked out, as well as my plan, and quickly realized my official training needed to start next week.

I dusted off the rainbow warrior and filled the flat tires with air in order to take it out on its maiden voyage. I had only gone about three miles when both tires became flat. What I failed to recognize was the tires and tubes were dry rotted. I had also failed to bring my cellphone and had no way of contacting Jacki for a ride home. I did not want to leave the rainbow warrior on the side of the road fearing it would have been stolen. The only saving grace was the pedals on the bike had cages that you would insert your sneakers into as opposed to the fancier clip in pedals which utilized biking specific shoes. I hoisted the bike onto my shoulder and ran the three miles home trying to optimistically remind myself at least I was getting in some run training. The next day I purchased new tires and tubes for the bike as well as a small repair kit that sat in a bag underneath the seat.

The first week of training left me sore and tired. It also became very apparent to me that biking was my least favorite activity of the three and I was not incredibly good at it. To make matters worse I just never felt comfortable in the saddle. I did like that the training was all mapped out for me, and I only needed to do my best to follow it. There was no guess work. I stayed with it for the next two weeks and looked forward to the recovery week which would occur every fourth week.

After two months of training I saw that there was going to be a shorter triathlon in nearby Pittsford. I promptly signed up for the Pittsford Sprint Triathlon thinking it would be a good idea to experience racing in one and help me during my transitions from the swim to the bike and the bike to the run. This was where you needed to get into your biking gear after the swim and then change into your running attire after the bike. I also thought the shorter distance of the race which included a 300-yard pool swim, 15-mile bike and 3.3 mile run would be relatively easy. I would come to regret that line of thinking.

Race day came and I nervously waited in a line alongside the pool for my turn in the swim. I slipped into the pool and, after getting the go signal, pushed off the wall and began swimming as fast as I could. I needed to swim 12 lengths or six laps. After each lap you would go under the lane line and swim in the adjacent lane until you reached the far end of the pool. By my third lap I was feeling exhausted and must have looked like I was swimming as if I was on fire. I knew I was slowing down because the person behind me kept slapping the back of my feet with their hands. When I reached the next wall, I stayed there to let them go ahead of me. I didn't want to let go of the wall and realized I had let my nerves get the best of me. I had failed to pace myself. Upon exiting the pool I was breathing heavily as I ran across the parking lot to the transition area where my bike was staged.

I donned my socks, running shoes, shorts, and a shirt before walking my bike out of the transition area. I took off on the rainbow warrior while mentally reminding myself to not go all out. Up to this point all of my bike training had taken place around my house where there were no hills, and the roads were flat as a pancake. I soon discovered that the Pittsford-Mendon area was not like that, and the course had numerous hills. I remember at one point I was in my lowest gear and barely moving up what I thought to be a steep hill. My legs were burning with lactic acid and so much for not going all out. A ton of people passed me on my bike reinforcing my belief that biking was not my strong suit. I wanted to desperately reach the transition area so that I could start the run and get off this torture chamber.

Eventually I arrived at the transition area and placed my bike in the rack. As soon as I stepped away from it, I was surprised that my legs felt like Jell-O and as if they weighed 100 pounds each. I had done "bricks" during training, meaning I would run after biking, but my legs never felt like this. I began jogging on the run course and immediately knew this was not going to be good. Luckily the first part of the run was downhill, and my legs started to feel better, but they were still heavy. On the backside of the run course was a long gradual hill that started to suck the life out of me. I had to fight exceptionally hard to quell the urge to walk because I was that tired. I'm fairly certain I saw a snail and a turtle pass me before reaching the top. I tried to go as fast as possible after that because I could hear the cheers from the finish line, but my legs just weren't cooperating. I remember reaching the finish line and instead of feeling happy and accomplished, I had a head full of negative thoughts that included, *"Why was this so hard? Maybe all the experts were right, and I'm way in over my head."*

It was a somber ride home because I knew once again, I was at a crossroads. I knew I had two choices-walk back my plans of being an Ironman that year or stop feeling sorry for myself and forge a new path ahead. It wasn't that I had done horribly in the race and came in last. I finished 101 out of 267 racers. The thing that got me was how hard the race was and how bad I felt during it. The one thought that was difficult to shake was it took me 1 hour and 37 minutes to do that race and I knew an Ironman would take me at least 12 hours to complete. I wrestled with that thought all day. Luckily,

I had also thought about my SWAT brothers, Wemo, Tommy Valentine, and my sons who knew I had already committed to doing an Ironman. I decided I would stay the course but with a new perspective.

Through much soul-searching I had realized while I was training the last two months, I was merely going through the motions, completing the training sessions, and not fully applying myself. It was considered a win to merely complete the distances. My new commitment would be to try and find a better me during every training session. This did not mean I would go all out 110% during the entire session but rather strategically pick points during the sessions and hang on for dear life. This might mean running an eight-minute mile for one mile during a 10-mile training run or maintaining a 19 mph speed on the bike for two miles out of a 30-mile ride. I needed to do this to bulletproof my mind so I could fight back the negative self-talk or what I had labeled as demons. Plain and simple I needed to be mentally tougher and was hoping this would accomplish that.

I started the next training block with this new mentality and a fresh set of lenses. It was certainly harder, both mentally and physically, to train this way but slowly over time I felt calluses forming on my soul. The training would open fresh wounds in my head and my heart. I would fight like hell to get past self-imposed barriers. These micro victories would cause those wounds to heal, and it was all that scar tissue I could look back on during difficult times in future trainings. Make no mistake about it, I would break at times during these sessions, and I tried to optimistically put that into perspective. My training goals were indeed hard to achieve. I stopped feeling disappointed about these failings and instead became pissed off. I used them as logs in the next training session to fuel the fire I felt in my soul. It was my first attempt at using bad or negative emotions to my advantage. Most of us instinctively know how to effectively use good and positive emotions to motivate ourselves and this was a huge paradigm shift for me. It was the start of a process that would allow me to discover a better understanding of what I was made of. A mindset that would later allow me to discover personal greatness.

A month later I entered another sprint triathlon sponsored by the Buffalo Triathlon Club. It was held at YMCA Camp Kenan on the shores of Lake Ontario. I had attended this camp numerous times as a youth and it felt like a homecoming. The triathlon had a law enforcement team division that had been dominated by the Niagara County Sheriff Department's team for the first two years. Coincidentally, my lifetime friend and best man at my wedding, Jim Hildreth, was a member of that team. I was on the RPD team with Kevin Chartrand and Aaron Colletti. They were both more experienced at triathlons than me and much better athletes. My biggest fear was letting them down. Another coworker, Kirk Pero, participated in the triathlon but you could only have three people on the team. I remember him jokingly threaten that none of us better finish behind him in the race.

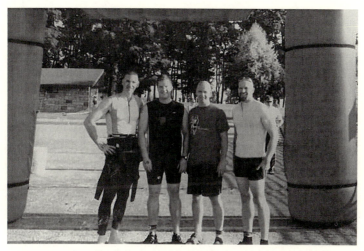

Kevin Chartrand, Kirk Pero, me, and Aaron Colletti at the sprint triathlon

I had what I would consider a very good race and my new mindset was paying off. A few negative thoughts popped into my head during the bike portion, but I quickly used them to stoke the flames inside of me. I had grown accustomed to running on unsteady legs after the bike and not a single person passed me on the run. Both of my teammates beat me, but I wasn't that far behind Aaron. We ended up winning the law enforcement division and took home a large trophy that I had engraved with our names on one of the empty nameplates. The idea was the trophy would be brought back the following year for the next race.

Unfortunately, the race was permanently canceled, and that trophy sat on my office shelf at work until I retired. It now prominently rests on a table in my living room. On an incredibly sad note, Aaron was struck and killed by a motorist while out bike riding with one of his sons on June 11th, 2020. It broke my heart to receive that news.

I went back to training realizing my new mentality was beginning to change me. I knew I wasn't bulletproof yet, but I was tougher than when I started. I still had anxiety about the length of the Ironman race and would often talk with Kevin about it. His message always remained the same. That it's hard to wrap your brain around it until you actually do one and after you will see things differently. It wasn't that I didn't believe him, but I couldn't comprehend what he meant.

After another month I found myself doing one more race before my Ironman. It was the Cayuga Lake Triathlon, an Olympic distance race that consisted of a .93-mile swim, 24.8 mile bike and 6.2 mile run. It was roughly twice the distance of a sprint triathlon. At Kevin's urging, I bought a used Trek Equinox triathlon specific bike that was a major upgrade from the rainbow warrior. It was considerably lighter due to its alloy frame and had more gears.

While I always had and will continue to have pre-race jitters, they weren't nearly as bad before this race. I was gaining confidence in my racing abilities even though I was nowhere close to placing in the top three of my age group. I was still that middle-of-the-pack guy and gray.

I swam straight and strong to start the race and became proficient at transitioning to the bike. Once on the bike, I was faced with a very steep hill that seemed to go on forever. Before long I was in my lowest gear and out of the saddle trying to turn each peddle over. The demons started spewing things like "You're going to stall and fall over," and "You might as well walk your bike." Even though I was working as hard as I could, I still managed to shoot them a small smile while internally saying, "Fuck off, I got this!" Once making it to the top I settled into a groove on my new bike. It made me faster but not nearly as much as I hoped it would. It was slightly more comfortable though. Before I knew it, I was flying down the same steep hill heading back to the transition area. As my speed approached 40 mph, I began pumping my brakes while other Kamikaze riders passed me like I was standing still. It was the most scared I have ever been on a bike and was relieved to pull into the transition area to begin the 10-kilometer run.

The demons in my legs immediately began acting up but I told them there was no place for them in my body. The farther I ran the faster I got. I vowed that no one would pass me. At the Taughannock Falls, which was only a trickle due the exceptionally dry summer, I was halfway into the run and now heading back to the finish line. The demons had long exited my legs and not another one spoke to me. I crossed the finish line feeling proud, accomplished, and fierce.

I used that race to springboard into my final three weeks of incredibly long training sessions. Biking was still my Achilles heel, but I had become better at it. I was very comfortable in the water and had convinced myself Poseidon was surely in my family lineage. Running was still my "strong" suit and I had been training at a 10-minute mile pace on my long runs to include a 22 miler. I asked Kevin if it would be possible to maintain that running pace during the race and he politely told me no. As much as I respected him, I chose not to believe him. My other strong suit was I flourished in hot sticky weather. My mantra was the hotter the better because I never enjoyed training in a cold environment. While the oppressive sun would suck the life out of other triathletes, I felt like a solar panel, and it would recharge me. I knew the race in Maryland would be hot and it never really concerned me.

I made it through those three long weeks of training and each session was another callus. There was a failure here and there but again, it meant the training was meaningful. I was happy to begin the three week tapering process, meaning the training would gradually taper off so my body would recover and heal. For those who have never done tapering, it's a scary process. Mentally, you feel as if you are going to lose all your hard-fought gains and lose fitness. Physically, all types of weird aches and pains come to the surface as your body repairs itself. Luckily, I had an old friend who had completed numerous marathons and had keen insight on tapering. It was Lisa Cleary-Schroeder who I affectionately call, the "Marathon Queen." We had been good friends since high school, and she was a standout gymnast. She was truly my saving grace during this troubled time and kept me from going too hard. I needed to trust the training program the same way I trusted it in the buildup phase. While the sessions were shorter in length and duration, they also ramped up to a faster pace. The philosophy was to repair and rest the body while keeping the proverbial sword sharp.

It wasn't long before I found myself in Maryland along with Jacki and good friend Wayne. At the pre-race meeting we were told the conditions would be perfect for the race which was the following day. The race director explained that the tide would be going out of the Chesapeake Bay where we would be swimming and it would be as if we had a boat motor strapped to our feet. This made me feel optimistic because when I looked at the distances between the swim buoys it appeared to be much longer than 2.4 miles.

I didn't sleep much that night because of the anxiety I was feeling. While waiting to start the race I had a stomach full of butterflies and a very real fear of the unknown. It didn't help that a rogue storm came in and we would now be swimming in 1-to-2-foot waves for the entire length of the swim. *So much for being a fast swim*, I thought. The race started and I felt like I was swimming in a mosh pit. There were arms flying and feet kicking everywhere. I kept searching for unoccupied water but just couldn't find any for the first five minutes. After that we all began to spread out and I focused hard on maintaining a steady stroke. I would lift my head straight out of the water after a dozen or so strokes to make sure I was swimming straight towards the next buoy. I swam past buoy after buoy until I saw the exit area. I had spent almost an hour and a half in the water before entering the transition area to start the bike portion.

I quickly changed into my biking gear and was out on the road tackling the 112-mile bike ride. Most of the bike course consisted of completing two loops through the Black Water National Refuge. The good part about the course was the roads were flat just like back home. The bad part was a steadily blowing wind and no matter which way I was going, I felt like it was always in my face. The downside to a flat windy course is that you can never stop peddling, or you will quickly slow to a stop. Numerous times I would round a corner and there would be Jacki and Wayne shaking cowbells and cheering me on. That would always bring a huge smile to my face even though I was suffering on the inside on what I always describe as a torture chamber, my bike. I tried to stay in the aero position meaning my elbows resting on pads on the handlebars while my hands gripped forward-facing handlebar extensions. This would cause me to hunch over in a tucked position to minimize aerodynamic drag. One of the downsides is you needed to crane your neck up in order to see down the road. I tried hard in training to embrace this position however, I would find myself constantly going between it and riding upright.

I began the second loop feeling somewhat dejected because the winds became stronger, and I was feeling more fatigued. It didn't help that I had not passed a single soul; however, I was passed numerous times by other racers. I fought hard against the demons that were raging in both my body and mind but never to the point where I felt like quitting. I just wanted to get off that damn bike and start the 26.2 marathon run. I soon began to smell a heavy stench of smoke in the air but did not see a fire. I had later learned that part of the refuge began to burn, and I had just made it past that area before they diverted the racers behind me onto another road, thus shortening their bike portion. Later I would often joke that I wish I would have been that lucky.

I was never so happy to see the high school where I transitioned from the bike to the run. After changing out of my biking shoes and into my running sneakers I began to run onto the course while constantly telling myself, *You knew it was going to be like this. You knew it was going to be like this.* "This" was that my legs were extremely heavy and unsteady. I also knew I just needed to run a few miles to bring them back to life. The run portion consisted of three loops and the race finished on the high school track. It had been a clear day, and by this time the sun was really beating down with temperatures well into the 80s. I may have been the only racer that thought it felt great. I just knew I had to continually drink to stay hydrated in such hot weather.

Soon my legs felt much better, and I settled into a familiar 10-minute mile race pace with that conversation with Kevin looming in the background of my brain. Mile after mile I started to feel stronger and stronger. I would admittedly walk away from each aid station while drinking a cup full of Gatorade or water. Once it was finished, I would begin running again.

Upon finishing my first lap and passing by the high school, I saw Jacki and Wayne cheering me on. They had now been joined by Katie Hibbard who is still a great friend of mine. To this day she still calls me "Ironman" which always puts a big smile on my face. I had met Katie and her husband Jeff the night before at race check-in and learned they were from Hilton, a neighboring village where I lived. I was slightly jealous because the three of them, along with waving cowbells, were drinking ice cold beer and wine coolers. I continued running along at a 10-minute mile pace and even faster at times. A new phrase started repeating in my brain, *You are doing it.* I was in the late stages of a race that nearly seemed impossible a short six months ago. I tried not to think too far ahead because I knew I still had almost three hours of running to do, but it helped that now I was doing the passing, and no one had passed me. I had started to make up ground on Jeff who was several miles ahead of me, and every time we passed by each other he would joke, "You're catching me."

While beginning the third and final loop, I suddenly felt myself approaching the breaking point. There were numerous blisters forming on my feet and several toenails began to loosen. As much as I loved the sun, I could feel myself starting to fry. I could also feel extreme tightness in my calves as if they were about to ball up and seize at any moment. The emotions I began to feel now were the bad ones -- fear, sorrow, and self-pity. I tried hard to use them as fuel, but I was not fully accomplished at that task yet. I felt my pace beginning to slow and thought maybe Kevin was right, I can't maintain a 10-minute mile pace through the run. For all intents and purposes, I had rapidly hit rock bottom and the demons were winning. I then began to feel the emotions of anger and rage and directed them at the course. It came out of nowhere but was the beginning of an enlightenment process, realizing that the course was a living entity. Its purpose was to inflict pain upon me and to impede my progress in finishing. It became my only adversary and I stopped thinking about the runners that were in front of me. I became full of fury directed at the pavement I was running on. I wanted to hurt it, not with my fists, but with my feet. Each foot strike was a win for me and a loss for it. I stopped thinking about my pace and only about doling out punishment. I was still hanging by a thread, but this gave me a reason not to break. I then took it a step further.

I noticed the sun was much lower in the sky and I laid down the challenge, I would finish while it was still daylight. I further added that finishing in the dark would mean the course had won. I constantly beat back demons that would barrage me with things like, "It's not gonna hurt if you just walk for a little bit." And, "It doesn't matter if you finish in the dark, you'll still be a finisher." I knew these were lies and would try to summon more rage and fury. I had never been turned this far inside out and there was nowhere to hide. Every emotion was raw, primal, and real, and what startled me was I liked it. Nothing was fake or superficial, the way we often are when going through the motions of everyday life. As I approached the finish line, I looked over my shoulder and a quarter of the sun was still above the tree line. My immediate thought was, *I fucking won!*

I was quickly met by Jacki and Wayne and all those raw emotions of rage, fear, and fury left me. The moment I crossed the finish line, those emotions were instantly replaced with joy and a pronounced feeling of accomplishment. Physically I was a wreck and could barely stand. I just wanted to stop moving however I began experiencing vertigo whenever I remained motionless. Everything between my teeth and toes was in distress and while I tried to embrace it, I felt myself shying away from it. I was extremely happy to have finished in a little over 12 1/2 hours, but I had never felt like this physically. I didn't want to drink or eat anything, I just wanted to feel better. I averaged 10:02 minute miles on the run and should have been happy but I couldn't stop thinking I was 52 seconds over what I was shooting for.

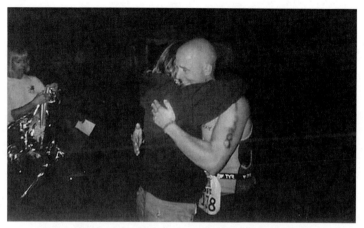

A congratulatory hug from Jacki at the finish of the
Chesapeakeman triathlon

The recovery process took the better part of three months. A certain pain would begin to fade and a new one would take its place. I couldn't run and certainly wasn't getting back on my bike. I would go for the occasional swim to try loosening my tight and sore body. Once I finally got back to a regular training routine, I noticed something had changed. It wasn't an A-ha moment, but I began looking at things through a different lens. The anticipation of particularly hard training days no longer made me stressed. Difficult SWAT training days became easier. I truly believe turning myself inside out during both the training and the actual race, changed my perspective on hardship. As much as it had hurt, a small part of me missed it because it was so real and true. I learned much about myself during that process and knew I had more to discover.

The following year I entered every triathlon in Western NY with most of them being sprint or Olympic distances. Aaron Colletti told me about a race he had been trying to get into for the past two years called Escape from Alcatraz. It consisted of a 1.5-mile swim that started off a ferry adjacent to the island the famous Alcatraz Prison sits on. The water in the San Francisco Bay was bitterly cold and the outgoing tide would drag swimmers out to the ocean if they did not account for it. Once exiting the water I would have to run a half mile to my bike. I was told it wasn't always this way but after numerous bike crashes due to racers having numb fingers from the swim, and unable to manipulate their bike brakes, the run was added to warm up the athletes. There was hardly a flat portion to the 18-mile bike ride. If you weren't going up, then you were going down. The race culminated with an eight-mile run under the Golden Gate Bridge which included deep sands and a 400-step sand ladder up a steep cliff. I was instantly intrigued and put in for the lottery. Aaron had also put in for the third time.

A month later Aaron and I were at our respective work desks when he yelled over to me that once again, he did not get into the race. I immediately checked my email and learned I was accepted! After re-reading it a couple times, I yelled back to Aaron that I had gotten in. He could tell from my voice that I was telling the truth and jokingly responded, "I hate you." I promptly returned, "I love you too Aaron!"

I really enjoyed doing the race that summer. The terrain made it especially difficult, and I had learned firsthand why no escaped inmates could make that swim. It was my hardest swim to date because of the freezing water and strong tides. I was never so happy to feel dry land under my feet upon exiting the water.

In 2009, I returned to longer training days in preparation for the Louisville Ironman. I was still seeing things differently and no longer did the thought of a 22-mile run or 100-mile bike ride keep me up at night. I slept contently knowing I had been through this fire and came out intact. Once again Wayne made the trip along with Jacki. I bested my time by 15 minutes over my Maryland race with the Louisville bike course being much more difficult. The toll on both my body and brain had been about the same though. The picture of me hunched over, leaning against a building after that race sums things up pretty well. I was in quite a bit of distress and couldn't walk because my calves and hamstrings had seized due to cramping.

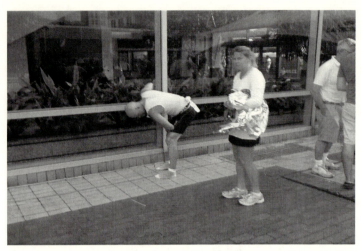

15 minutes after finishing the Louisville Ironman race

Friends, family, and coworkers who knew of my training and races would often jokingly ask, "What's next?" I didn't have a specific answer other than I planned to do more triathlons. All of this would change after a seemingly harmless conversation with a Drug Enforcement Agency (DEA) agent I knew.

Chapter 7- The Point of No Return

I crossed paths with DEA Special Agent Brian Hanley in the early summer of 2010, after attending a meeting at his office. He was a man of shorter stature with a muscular build and a laid-back style. I would have guessed him to be a surfer. He and his work partner, DEA Special Agent Jim Schmitz, had run the Rochester Marathon together a year earlier. During the race they crossed paths with Jacki who was also running the race. They ran with her for the rest of the race and kept her in good spirits. Brian told me he was doing the Beast of Burden 24-hour Ultra Marathon race in August. I had never heard about ultra-marathons and was instantly intrigued. What was even more interesting was the racecourse was on the Erie Canal towpath and started in my hometown of Lockport. Brian said he would be running 12.5 miles to Middleport then back to Lockport. He would try to run as many loops as possible during the 24 hours. What he said next would eventually change my life. Thank you, Brian! He explained after the first 25 miles he was allowed to have "pacers" run with him and keep him company. He asked if I was interested in helping him and I couldn't resist.

I worked overtime the day of the race and returned home well past midnight. After picking up Jacki, we headed for Middleport where we would eventually meet up with Brian. It was raining when I pulled into the parking lot and first noticed the headlamps and blinking lights the racers were wearing. Some were running and others were walking hunched over like zombies. Even through the rain I could see the suffering in their faces. I thought it was remarkable!

Brian showed up around 3 am and I was going to run with him first. He was in good spirits for being 62 ½ miles into the race. We began to speed walk west on the canal path. We walked and walked until I couldn't bite my tongue any longer. I asked when we were going to run, and he explained he ran the first part of the race and was now making good time speed walking. What he said next hit me like a double dare bet, that most people can't run the entire race and will eventually end up walking a good part of it.

We continued to walk until the town of Gasport where Jacki and I switched. I drove the car to Lockport and waited for them to arrive. The sun was just beginning to rise as they rolled into Lockport. Brian was limping a little and said he needed to soak his feet in ice water. When he took his socks off his feet looked like they had gone through a meat grinder. They were red, full of blisters and badly swollen. There was something eerily fascinating about it, that it was earned through the will to continue to push forward. He knew he wouldn't make it all the way back to Middleport before the end of the race but was going to see how far he could go.

We wished him well and started our drive home. I kept thinking about his words regarding walking and I couldn't stop it from looping in my head. Eventually

I told Jacki what he said and without a shed of proof, I said I thought I could run the race. She gave me the "oh no" look and shook her head. She wasn't doubting me but knew I was contemplating doing the race. While I had completed two marathons during my Ironman races, I had never run a stand-alone marathon because it just never appealed to me.

A week after the race Brian gave me the book, *Ultramarathon Man- Confessions of an All-night Runner* by Dean Karnazes, as a thank you. Once I started reading it, I couldn't put it down. It was full of suffering, personal growth, and transformation. Karnazes helped to popularize ultra-marathons through his various feats and books. Between the book and my time spent with Brian during his race, I was hooked. The next adventure was the Beast of Burden 100 Mile Ultra Marathon on August 20th, 2011.

I researched everything there was on training and racing ultra-marathons and developed my own 7 1/2 month training schedule. Each week included a longer run followed the next day by a "backup" run which was half the distance of the long run. This would help to boost my endurance but more importantly had me running on sore tired legs that replicated the later stages of a race. There were two other runs each week as well as a day of swimming and another of biking. The long runs would increase a mile each week and every fourth week was a recovery week were I would cut back the mileage. My longest run was 30 miles which was followed by a three week taper. I experimented during every long run with nutrition and hydration. Success in races this long is won and lost by what you put in your body during them. I would soon put that to the test and my goal was to finish the race in under 24 hours.

On April 17th, I ran the BPAC Ultra in Buffalo, NY which was a six hour race. It was a cold windy day, and I was nervous because my longest training run had only been 13 miles. Jacki, Zachary, and Wayne would provide me with food and drink every time I returned from a three mile loop. I ran the entire six hours and completed 32.5 miles. I was sore and fatigued after and had flash-backs to the Pittsford Triathlon. I only went a third of the distance of the Lockport race and felt I didn't have an-other mile left in me. I had that "over my head" feeling yet again, coupled with trying to wrap my brain around running 100 miles. Still I progressed with my training with a "So let it be written, so let it be done" attitude. I needed to follow my plan.

A coworker, Investigator Bill Lawler, was an avid marathoner and had recently been diagnosed with Huntington's disease. I thought someone should benefit from my race and approached him about raising money for a local Huntington's disease research organization he supported. He enthusiastically accepted my offer.

A short time later, Sergeant Bill Mahoney, another coworker, unexpectedly fell ill and passed away leaving behind a wife and three children. I had known Billy since he came on the job and there wasn't a nicer man. I knew

I wanted to also do something for his family without re-neging on the other Bill. I decided on "Running for the Bills" and the donations would be split down the middle.

Most of the donations came from police officers and a local radio personality had heard about my plans. It was Bob Lonsberry, who was an avid marathoner. Years before he had worked as a reporter for a local newspaper and did a story involving one of my near-death incidents. He invited me on his show, and we immediately hit it off. He has been a friend ever since and with his help I raised over $18,000.

Race day came and it was over 80° before the race started at 10 am. I barely slept the night before and anxiously paced while waiting for the race to start. It was then when Bill's wife, Jen and one of her children, unexpectedly showed up. We hugged and cried and most of my nerves went away.

When the race started, I fought the urge to go too fast and a majority of the other runners surged ahead of me. Jacki and Zachary would meet me every couple miles on the towpath to supply food and drink. I wasn't allowed to have pacers until completing the first loop and was surprised how much those first 25 miles taxed me.

My first pacer, SWAT brother Eric Alexander, led me out of Lockport. He kept running ahead of me while encouraging me to keep up. I had miscommunicated about his role and that I was the one to set the pace. I obliged and we ran much faster than I had planned.

Once in Middleport, SWAT brothers Herb McClellan and Brian Sexstone took over. They provided much needed encouragement and would run ahead to get me food and drink. Next up in Lockport was my mentor, Pete Brunett. I was hot and tired with my feet beginning to blister but his energy made all of that dull. SWAT brother Ryan Hickey switched with Pete in Middleport and helped to steady me because the wheels were starting to come off. My feet grew sorer with each step and giant rashes had formed on my inner thighs. I fought hard to make it back to Lockport where SWAT brother Todd Baxter waited to begin mile 75.

I knew I needed to clean my rashes and apply ointment to them. I asked my son Gabriel to get me the wet wipes I had packed for the race. He mistakenly grabbed the ones out Jacki's glovebox and those contained alcohol. In a public bathroom, I began wiping down the bloody rashes and instantly felt a stinging pain from the alcohol. I quickly placed my bare bottom in the sink and began splashing it with water to make the pain go away. Words cannot describe how bad it hurt.

After getting myself right, Todd and I started running and our conversation turned to Wemo. I had asked him to run with me but earlier that month a helicopter with 30 Americans, including 17 SEALS from Wemo's base, was shot down in Afghanistan killing all aboard. It is commonly referred to as Extortion 17. Todd and I agreed to dedicate the next 12 ½ miles to Wemo and his fallen brothers. Not a minute later, thick clouds and wind moved in, and the sky lit up with lightning. I had checked the forecast before the race, and this wasn't in it. My immediate thought was, "Oh shit, we woke those guys up!" Todd and I looked at each other but didn't say a word, we knew they were showing us some "love." Those warriors thrived on adversity and figured we could use a little more it. Across the canal a lightning bolt nearly touched down in a cornfield with a simultaneous ear deafening crack of thunder. Those boys were really getting rowdy! I jokingly thought Todd was screwed because he was five inches taller and would get struck before me. I also knew full well I would hug him if it happened, and we take that ride together. I relayed this incident to Wemo after the race and he agreed with my analysis. Due to this experience, the AC/DC song *Thunderstruck* was added to the other six songs on my running playlist.

As we ran into Middleport and, as if on cue, the clouds parted, the rain ended, and the stars came back out. SWAT brother Scott Peters would run the last 12 ½ miles with me. I was now hanging on by a thread and felt like someone had smashed both the tops and bottoms of my feet with sledgehammers. Blisters bulged on both feet and my toenails felt like they were on fire. My calves were hard as rocks and on the verge of seizing up. I couldn't fully embrace the suffering like I did during Ironman racing because this was at a whole new level.

It was a giant flame, and I was turning away from it instead of facing it.

At this point I was running for 15 minutes and walking for five with Scott keeping track of the time. The running minutes felt like hours while the walking breaks felt more like seconds. With six miles to go I sensed the thread unraveling and told Scott I needed a moment. In a sign of weakness, I placed my hands on my knees while bending over. My thoughts were cloudy, and I was desperately searching for a reason to continue. I felt a gentle hand on my shoulder and when I looked up, I saw Billy Mahoney. He told me I could do it and it felt like getting struck by lightning. When I up-righted myself, he was gone. It felt very real and made me both happy and sad. I struggled to start walking and slowly began to run. Earlier in the race each mile felt like a small victory and now it was each step. The sun had already risen well before we reached Lockport.

The course travels past the finish line on the other side of the canal for a mile before doubling back after crossing a bridge. It was at that 98-mile mark when I looked across the canal and saw Zachary knocking on Todd's car window. He had slept in his car after pacing me for 12 ½ miles. Todd emerged from the car with a stiffened gate, and I laughed to myself thinking he looked as bad as I did. He then began paralleling us.

Scott and I finally reached the bridge with one mile to go. Todd met us on the other side and had loosened up his tight legs. Out of nowhere a pickup truck skidded to a stop on the wrong side of the road and Ryan, Eric and Brian piled out and began running with us. They had spent the night in Niagara Falls and didn't think I would finish this quickly. The band was back together, and I fed off their brotherhood and love for me. Slowly I began to run faster and faster. I remember Todd asking me in disbelief, "What the hell you doing, Sobieraski?" Together we pushed the pace down to a 7:30 minute mile with my sons now joining us. We all crossed the finish line as a team in 21 hours and 52 minutes. I was officially an ultra-marathoner.

We all briefly celebrated, and I could tell everyone was tired. The race director, Sam Pasceri, presented me with a finisher's belt buckle which is a common prize for completing these races. He was surprised this was my first ultra because he said I looked strong the entire race and couldn't believe I finished in under 22 hours. I certainly didn't feel I had a strong race. He went on to ask me how far my drive home was and explained that in an hour or two things might get a little weird. Sam said I would experience tremors, chills and shallow breathing as my body begins to regulate itself. I hadn't read about any of this during my research.

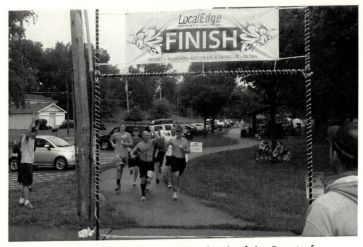

Wayne cheering us on at the finish of the Beast of
Burden 100 miler

Upon arriving home I shuffled into the shower and
the water rinsed the crusted sweat from my body directly onto my bloody rashes. The pain nearly brought me
to my knees. I crawled into bed and just wanted to fade
away. It hurt just to exist and then it started -- uncontrollable shaking and shallow breathing. Sam was right!
Jacki came in the bedroom and began to panic when she
saw my condition. I reminded her what Sam had said
but she was still nervous. After 30 minutes things im-
proved, and I so wanted to sleep but couldn't.

I managed to drag myself to work the next day
but had to wear slide sandals because my swollen feet
wouldn't fit into any of my shoes. I wore a size 9 running shoe that was a 1/2 size bigger than my feet. I later
learned it's better to go up 1-1 1/2 sizes to accommodate

for the foot swelling that occurs during ultras. This helped me tremendously in the future.

Thirty-five runners did not finish (DNF) the race. I'm guessing it was because of the weather. It had reached 92° that day with high humidity and not a cloud in the sky during the day. Twenty-eight did finish and I came in seventh place reaffirming I still had gray in me. What amazed me was the first place finisher ran it in 17 hours 52 minutes. He looked like he was running a 5k the entire time and I wasn't sure how that was possible.

It took me a full four months to recover from the race. I once again gained a new perspective when it came to hardship. I now feared very little of it. I knew what it was like to hit rock bottom and continue on. I also wondered if the elevator had truly run out of floors on the way down and I felt a strong need to answer that question. I was proud of my accomplishment but felt I could do better. I didn't feel personal greatness because I still had not stared down that flame.

I wasn't fully sure what to make of my Billy Mahoney experience during the race because it felt so real. Several years later I had a similar experience. After a small party at our house, I had my son Zachary drive me 10 miles down the road. I needed to do a 20 mile run the next day and about every three miles I instructed him to pull over. I would then stash either a large bottle of Gatorade or two bottles of water in the high grass near telephone poles. Admittedly hungover and dehydrated the next day, I began the run in 90° sticky weather. I reached the first bottle of Gatorade and nearly drank the entire thing. I continued on and, much to my dismay, I couldn't find the next set of water bottles. After an exhaustive search, I moved on. The location of the Gatorade bottle at mile 10 was now within sight and I couldn't believe what happened next. A man on a riding lawnmower came out of nowhere and headed towards the ditch where I stashed the bottle. The next thing I heard was the grinding of the mower blades on the bottle and red liquid sprayed from the mower deck. I disappointedly turned and headed for home knowing I was physically in trouble.

As much as I loved hot weather, I felt myself cooking. I again searched for the water bottles, but it was in vain. At this point I had stopped sweating and knew I needed to get home soon. I ran as hard as I could to the next Gatorade bottle and drank the little amount that was left. I had now developed a severe headache and was experiencing heat exhaustion. My body wanted to lie down but I knew I needed to get home.

The harder I ran, the more dizzy I became, and then the dry heaves started. I was still two miles from my house and fading fast. This was the exact point where it happened. I saw Fran's face and he told me, "You can make it home." He left as quickly as he had appeared. I remember tears running down my face as I ran as fast as I could. I didn't stop until I reached my bathroom, getting in a cold shower while drinking the water that fell upon me and quietly thanking Fran.

These experiences were confusing to me until it was explained in terms I could understand. Bob Lonsberry agreed to let me run with him during a trail marathon in 2021 and I told him of my encounters with those who have died. He is one of the most insightful people I know and explained that by me suffering so much, the veil between this life and the next had become paper thin allowing me to pierce it. It suddenly all made sense. To me it was the greatest benefit I received from soul stealing suffering. The ability to deeply connect with those I missed the most. I eagerly sought out these moments even though they were few and far between.

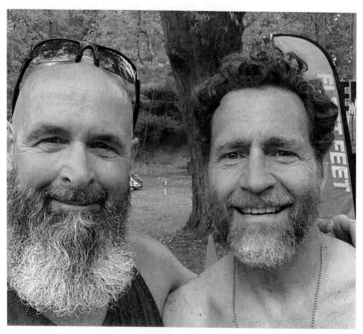

With Bob Lonsberry after we finished the Sehgahunda
Trail Marathon

Lastly, my heart felt different after the Beast of Burden race. I was still greatly saddened by Fran's passing and would often think of him while training. During many of my runs I would have one-way conversations with him. I would tell him of my family and work and that I missed him. I acknowledged that I had a form of PTSD and there was no answer as to why he died so young. I had eventually settled on the belief that bad things happen to good people and life is not fair. I was finally beginning to heal. There was still a giant hole in my heart, but I noticed it was starting to fill in with the love for my SWAT brothers. I trusted them with my life and our bond was forged through hardship and brotherhood. Whether it was during training and missions or through racing. They weren't replacing Fran but rather filling the void he had left. Many years later I eventually told my brothers of Fran at a private SWAT party they hosted for my retirement. It was the first time I had talked to them about him, and I needed them to know how much they meant to me and what they had done for me. Long Live the Brotherhood.

Chapter 8- A Glimpse of Personal Greatness

I inadvertently came across an advertisement for moisturizing eye drops and their front man was no other than Sam Pasceri, the race director for the Beast of Burden. I believe the company also sponsored his race. The ad listed many of Sam's impressive endurance accomplishments with one being a Double Ironman. I had no idea what that was, so the research began. Thank you, Sam!

The race was officially called the Double Anvil because the Ironman Corporation forbade them from using their trademarked name. I had initially thought one would do back-to-back Ironman's, but the race simply doubled the distances- 4.8 mile swim, 224 mile bike and 52.4 run. As insane as it sounded, I couldn't stop thinking about it. I stopped thinking and signed up for the October 2013 race.

I used the framework from my old Ironman training plan and added "backup" days after every long swim, bike and running day. I knew going into this it would be my longest race as it relates to distance and time and set to finish in 29 hours or under as my goal.

The training was brutal, and I developed patellar tendinitis in both my knees. I continued to train while attending physical therapy sessions although they wanted me to rest. There was no way I wasn't going to do the race and I hoped the eventual tapering process would allow my patellae to repair themselves.

Jacki and Wayne were going to be my crew and we all left for Virginia. They set up a pop-up canopy tent which would serve as my aid station along the race route in Lake Anna State Park.

The swim was lap after lap around buoys in Lake Anna. I still felt Poseidon's blood pulsing through my veins and came out of the water feeling great after over 2 1/2 hours of straight swimming. That would quickly change. The bike course was 2.5 miles long with traffic cones you had to loop around at each end. I needed to do 45 laps. It was mind numbing especially since I still didn't enjoy being on the bike and, to make matters worse, it rained most of the time. I spent over 15 hours on the torture chamber and only left the saddle three times to urinate. When I handed it off to Wayne, I remember telling him to burn it and I really meant it. I have only ridden that bike four times since.

I changed into running gear and it had been dark for hours. The run course was the same road as the bike, but you would only run out a mile and return for each loop. I needed to do 26 of these. I left the tent feeling like each leg carried an extra 25 pounds of lactic acid. The demons told me this was going to be bad and then it got worse. A mile into the third loop I felt like I was being stabbed in my right patellar tendon. The pain stopped me in my tracks and caused me to walk the remainder of that loop. Many thoughts went through my head during that time and most of them said my race was over. I hung on to a small sliver of rage I felt. I kept telling myself, *No fucking way! I wasn't going to DNF.* I made it back to the tent and both Jacki and Wayne knew I was in a bad way. I swallowed four ibuprofen tablets and defiantly left the tent. I kept trying to will the pain away and slowly I began to run. It was still painful, but I refused to walk. Eventually it dulled some and to this day I don't know if it was my willpower or the ibuprofen. My best guess was a combination of both.

I vowed no one would pass me and I kept that promise. On my last lap I proudly flew one of my SWAT Team's flags and crossed the finish in 29 hours 2 minutes. I was thankful I had overcome my knee issue but those damn two minutes still haunt me! It was a whole new level of discomfort after the race, and I almost couldn't walk the next day.

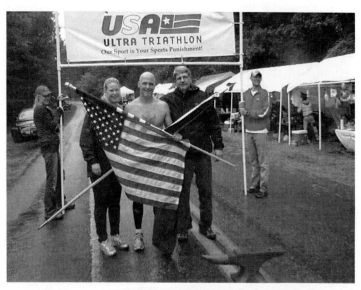

Jacki, me, and Wayne after finishing the Double Anvil triathlon in Virginia

While on the mend, Jacki walked in the house carrying a DVD she had rented. A running friend told her about the movie, *Running on the Sun: The Badwater 135,* and thought I would like it. It was a documentary about what has been dubbed "the world's toughest foot race."

Badwater 135 is a 135-mile ultra-marathon through California's Death Valley. The race starts in Badwater Basin, 280 feet below sea level, and finishes at an elevation of 8360 at the Whitney Portal, the trailhead to Mt Whitney, the highest mountain in the contiguous United States. The race crosses two other mountain ranges and temperatures have reached 130 degrees.

We watched it that night and I was instantly mesmerized by the sheer willpower of the runners and their collective sufferings. The next day I watched it twice. Thank you, Jacki! I knew I needed to do the race and began the research. Much to my dismay, I learned I needed to complete at least three 100 mile ultras. The application also included several essays that needed to be written. It noted that the proven ability to race in hot weather was a plus.

I scoured the internet for 100 mile ultras and found one in the Florida Keys. As a bonus, the race director of Badwater 135, Chris Kostman, was going to be participating as part of a relay team. I quickly signed up and began training after my wounds from the Double Anvil healed. Zachary made the trip to Florida with me and was my only crew. I would have no pacers. He pleasantly surprised me by spelling "SWAT Tough" on the side of our rented minivan with blue masking tape.

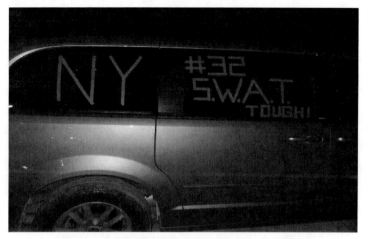

Our race vehicle for the Keys 100 ultra-marathon

It was an extremely hot race day, but I embraced the sun until I couldn't. At mile 42, I met up with Zachary for some Gatorade. My internal radiator was about to boil over so I sat in the passenger side of the minivan. I yelled at him to turn the air conditioning up high, and he laughed saying it was. The cold air coming out of the vents felt lukewarm at best. After five minutes he finally kicked me out of the van, and I felt as stiff as a board. My parting words to him was to never let me do that again.

After running another 12 miles I felt a stinging pain in my left pinky toe. I was pretty sure I knew what it was and tried my best to ignore it until it became almost unbearable. We stopped in the parking lot of an apartment complex and, after removing my shoe, my fear was confirmed. I had developed a blister on the end of my toe, and it forced the toenail to face straight up. Each stride caused the back of the toenail to be pushed deeper into my toe.

I popped the blister with a small needle, but the toenail would not lie back down. Not having a knife, I resorted to pulling the toenail off but there was one problem, the skin covering the end of my toe came with it. I threw the skin, with the still attached toenail, toward Zachary and the toe immediately began bleeding. He asked, "What the hell are you going to do now?" I shot him a hell-if-I-know look and had him get the medical box. I put a few band-aids on it and wrapped them with duct tape. My toe was now throbbing like it had its own pulse.

I began running and the pain was bearable, but I soon felt a weird sensation in my left sneaker. I kept telling myself to not look down but eventually my curiosity got the better of me. The left side of my white sneaker had turned red with blood and each time I looked down there was more red. I was worried because I still had 47 miles to run but stayed positive by assuring myself that no one had ever bled to death from their pinky toe.

Zachary snapped a picture of me around mile 90. I looked at it after the race and for the first time I noticed the "look." It is one of bewilderment, suffering and blankness all rolled into one. I jokingly refer to it as the near-death look, and I began to observe in other runners. To an extent it often mirrors how my soul feels and it's hard to hide anything when you are turned inside out.

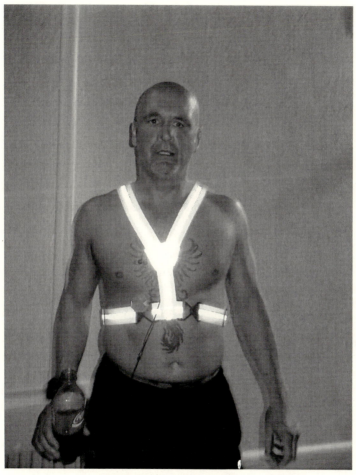

The "near death" look at mile 90 of the Keys 100

The race felt different because my SWAT brothers weren't there, but Zachary did a tremendous job and kept me in good spirits. I crossed the finish line in 19 hours and 12 minutes beating my Lockport time by over 2 1/2 hours. I knew my improvements were much more the result of mindset and mental conditioning than physical training. I was beginning to stare down the flame that only a year ago would make me turn away.

The other person who wasn't there was Jacki. We had decided on getting divorced earlier in the year. There was no midlife crisis, infidelity, or other nonsense. We just hadn't been getting along for some time. The process was amicable, and we used a mediator. She knew how important the house was to me and allowed me to stay there. I received the call from our mutual attorney the day after the race saying we were officially divorced. I had mixed emotions with most of them being sadness and a sense of failure. Upon returning home, we still lived together until she found a house of her own. My house was lonely after she left because it was just me, the boys were out on their own. Eventually I got used to the quietness and again, fully immersed myself in training.

Next up was round two of the Beast of Burden three months later. I assembled the same pacers with the addition of Aaron Springer and this time I raised money for the Veterans Outreach Center. Todd had become its Executive Director. My goal was to finish the race in under 18 hours which seemed absurd just three short years ago. At the starting line I prayed to be given the strength and courage of a United States veteran or in other words, the heart of a lion.

With my still progressing mental toughness, I ran hard but came to the crossroads at mile 50. I mismanaged my hydration on another blazing hot, humid day and developed cramps in my quadriceps and calves. I eventually hydrated and successfully willed them away. I also had help from another racer.

Every time I saw another competitor, I would say something encouraging such as, "Good job!" "Looking good!" or "Keep it up!" All would acknowledge my comments except for one lady. I realize we all suffer differently but every time I praised her, she would shoot me a mad look...every time! We crossed paths eight times during the race and after the fourth encounter, as petty as it may sound, I began using it to fuel me. At the halfway point she was up quite a few miles on me. Again, I'm sure she wasn't doing it on purpose but each time she snubbed me, I put another log on the fire.

As I neared the final turnaround point in Middleport on mile 88 ½, she was a half mile up on me. I picked up Ryan and Aaron and they would pace me to the finish line. They were both Army veterans and this provided even more logs for the fire. Just before reaching the Gasport aid station with roughly seven miles to go, I told them what food and drink I was going to get there and that I also needed to urinate in the porta potty. To my surprise I saw the lady sitting in a chair inside the aid station tent. I yelled to a perplexed Ryan and Aaron to get my stuff and catch up as I sped past the tent.

The two eventually caught me and gave me my supplies while asking what the hell was that about. For the first time, I openly voiced my displeasure towards the lady to them. By now we were running at a fast clip, and I was barely hanging on. I would catch Aaron constantly looking at me out of the corner of his eye to which I would think, *What the hell you looking at? I'm good to go.* That was partially a lie, and I knew he was looking out for me just like he did on SWAT. He now was the commanding officer of the Team.

I found myself intermittently asking them if she was behind us. They would look back and it went from, "I can see her headlamp," to "Looks like she's gaining on us," to "She's definitely getting closer." I refused to look back because I was confident it would cause me to stumble and fall. I thought I could almost hear her footsteps and braced for her passing. As we crossed the final bridge with one mile to go, I was able to glance over my shoulder and saw she was in fact over a quarter mile behind me. It was then I realized they had been lying to me and my initial thought was, *You bastards!* but they did what any good pacers should do. They provided me with motivation! In addition to that, Eric, Brian, and Pete joined in to finish the last mile with me.

I crossed the line in 18 hours and 44 minutes stealing third place from the "mean" lady. She crossed three minutes later and immediately approached me asking,

"How did you do that? How did you make up all that ground?" It almost sounded accusatory, but I knew it wasn't. I explained I don't fade as much as most racers. I wanted to also tell her that she should be a little nicer out on the course but didn't. She responded that what I had done was impressive and now she went from "mean" lady to "nice" lady.

I had fully embraced doing negative split training during all my runs and I believe it made me a better second half runner. By running each mile faster than the last in training, I had brainwashed my mind and body into going harder the more I tired. This is the exact opposite of what most do when running. No one would pass me after the midpoint of a race, but I would pass others. The training can be extraordinarily hard, but the dividends are well worth it.

I was disappointed I had finished 44 minutes over my goal time, but I was still heading in the right direction. This time was almost a half hour faster than my last race. I knew I was capable of going faster and, again, the key had to do more with training my brain than my body. My third place overall finish made me feel a lot less gray but to put matters in perspective, the winner beat me by 3 1/2 hours! Even so, I had a small taste of personal greatness, and I loved the feeling. I squarely faced the flame during this race and withstood its fury. The best part was I now had my three 100-mile races completed and could apply for the Badwater 135 race next year.

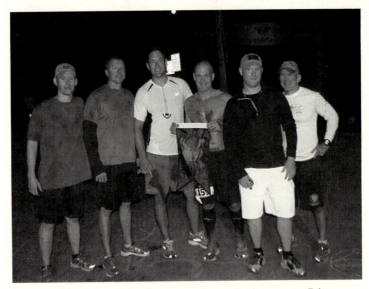

Ryan Hickey, Brian Sexstone, Aaron Springer, me, Eric Alexander, and Pete Brunett

Chapter 9- Full Steam Ahead

I eagerly awaited the application process to open for Badwater 135 in January 2015. I felt I had a decent chance of being accepted after showing I could race in the heat along with a strong finish in my last race. I wrote, rewrote, then revised the three essays I was required to submit. With a hope and a prayer I hit the send button.

A month later I received the Dear John email informing me I was not selected. It was a major disappointment and, after pouting for a few days, I began searching for a race to do that year. I came across the C&O Canal 100 ultra-marathon in Knoxville, Maryland. It resembled the Beast of Burden because the course was also on a canal path. The difference was the new race consisted of two loops and I wasn't allowed pacers until after 59 miles.

Five months earlier on September 3rd, 2014, RPD Officer Daryl Pierson was shot and killed while chasing a parolee. He left behind a wife and two young children. It not only devastated my department but the community as well. I had planned to do some sort of fundraiser for his family but by this time there had been plenty. I was told the family had grown weary of them. I still wanted to honor his memory and sacrifice, so I dedicated the race to him.

Ryan Hickey and Brian Sexstone would be my crew and pacers. They had both worked shoulder to shoulder with Daryl for many years in the Tactical Unit. Brian was still assigned with Daryl when was he murdered. My friend and coworker, Investigator John Fiorica, was the owner of Crime Dawg Inc. which made custom shirts. Free of cost, he made us shirts with my SWAT Team insignia on the left breast with a larger faded insignia on the back. Above that was "C&O Canal 100 Miler" and over the insignia were our names listed vertically with Office Pierson (EOW 9-3-14) being the first one. I called us Team Pierson.

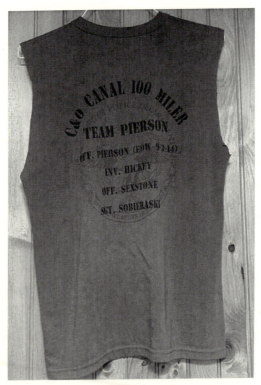

Team Pierson shirt

I only had nine weeks to prepare but had already been training in hopes of going to Death Valley. I just needed to ramp up the mileage and, more importantly, temper my mind. I didn't want to let Daryl down. To accomplish this I did most of my long runs on a treadmill at the YMCA. For me, nothing helps to build mental toughness more than running on a treadmill for hours on end. It's also a fail-proof way to train negative splits. Every mile I would raise the speed another .1 mph for the duration of the run.

Race day came quickly, and I stood at the starting line without the normal butterflies. I promised I would not allow myself to feel or be weak during the race so that no matter when Daryl looked down, he would be proud. Once again, my goal was to finish in under 18 hours.

At the 25-mile mark I felt extremely strong and was running faster than I should. Normally I would slow myself down but not that day, I didn't fight it. The next 29 miles dropped quickly and drama free except for some loosening toenails, rash, and a few blisters. After 59 miles Ryan and Brian took turns running with me and it was an instant motivator. This helped to counteract the rain and sleet that started right before nightfall. It continued for the rest of the race and completely flooded the course. It was mildly bothersome, but I was still running proud and strong.

At mile 90 it hit me that I couldn't feel anything emotionally. It was tough for me because I was used to running on emotions in the later stages of races. I knew I was inside out and more than I had ever been. Physically, I felt searing pain in my legs and feet. Spiritually, I began feeling the presence of a hero. Even though I didn't see him, it was still comforting, and I knew I was exactly where I needed to be.

I would catch my brothers looking at me out of the corner of their eyes. I could tell they knew I was hanging by a thread. But they also knew the unwritten SWAT rule about not breaking. We plowed ahead to a steep hill that included a stream crossing requiring us to step on rocks to cross it. This was followed by a series of switchbacks up the side of a ravine to the finish line. There was a racer ahead of me who was attempting to cross the stream while saying he could not see. He stepped on a rock and fell backwards. I caught him before he hit the ground and handed him off to Ryan as I jumped ahead. The clock was ticking. By now the path was slippery because of all the rain and I fell at least a half dozen times. Ryan caught up to me with Brian meeting us near the top. Team Pierson crossed the finish line together and a small part of me was sad the race was over.

Based on my "ranking" from my previous races, some computer program linked to the race had me finishing with a targeted time of 22 hours and 23 minutes. Team Pierson finished in 17 hours and 52 minutes. I had finally made my goal and felt supremely proud. I hoped Daryl felt the same and also knew SWAT brothers Ryan and Brian sacrificed much for me. If it wasn't for them,

I never would have completed in under 18 hours. Thank you, brothers!

From then on, the Team Pierson shirt I wore during the race would be worn during every SWAT mission until I retired. I looked at it as another form of armor keeping me safe. That now ragged shirt stands for brotherhood, perseverance and, most of all, the memory of a hero. I thought of his sacrifice every time I wore it.

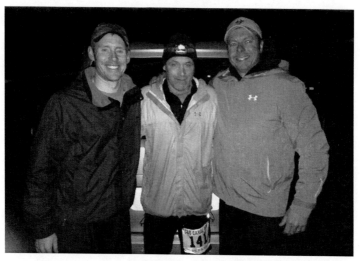

Team Pierson- Ryan Hickey, me (with the "near death" look) and Brian Sexstone

I had contemplated running the Beast of Burden for a third time that summer, but I had a few nagging ailments from the race. I was getting much better at re-covery, but something told me not to push it. My ride home every day took me right next to Lake Ontario. One day I looked across the lake and thought about Fran. He,

Paul, and I stayed in a cottage on the lake one summer and Fran and I would debate whether it was possible to swim across the lake to Toronto. It was a conversation that would pop up in my head every so often. I pulled my car over to the shoulder of the road and walked to the water. I thought to myself, *I wonder if I could do it?* I had no idea what the distance would be but that day I decided I was going to do it.

After some research I learned the "established" swim course was from Fort Niagara to Toronto with a distance of 32 miles. I didn't even know such a thing existed. There were even official rules and a governing organization if you wanted to be considered an "official finisher" and have your name added to the other 54 who had successfully swam it. I declined due to the cost. I felt the money would be put to better use by adding it to a fundraiser. I remembered Wemo telling me of Tommy Valentine's passing on February 13th, 2008, during High Altitude High Opening (HAHO) parachute training in Arizona at the age of 37. He was preparing for his 10th deployment in support of Operation Enduring Freedom and Operation Iraqi Freedom. He was a father, son, brother, and husband. He was also one of the most humble and genuine people I have ever met. Shortly after his death, his wife Christina created the All In, All The Time Foundation (AIATT) in his honor. The foundation fills the interim needs of surviving spouses and children of fallen Navy Special Warfare warriors. It alleviates some of the financial burdens, days, months, or years after the funeral. I dubbed my undertaking "Swimming for the Seals" with all of the proceeds going to AIATT.

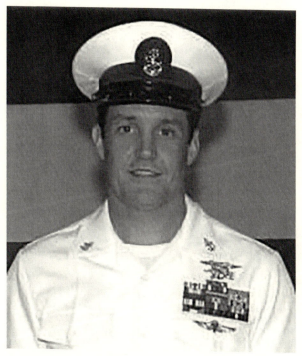

Senior Chief Petty Officer (SEAL) Thomas Valentine

I constructed my own training plan and tackled it much the same as my running plans by adding a backup day after weekly long swimming sessions. All of my early training swims were in the pool at the YMCA. Once the lake warmed my long swims would take place there. My longest swim was 7.5 miles, approximately a 1/4 of my swim distance to Canada. That swim was broken in half by a quick trip to the shore for some Gatorade. I nearly fell over upon standing and didn't know why. It also happened at the end of the swim. I later learned that being both horizontal and cold for that long, most of my blood was pooled in my core. This is what caused my imbalance and dizziness.

Based on my swim speed, I set the goal of finishing in less than 22 hours. I knew this would be particularly challenging especially since I had concerns about just finishing the swim. I could wrap my head around Ironman races and 100-mile ultra-marathons, but not this.

One of my other tasks was to find a boat to make the trip. Good friend and Colorado hunting mate, Jason Aymerich stepped up and borrowed a friend's boat. That guy always comes through in a pinch. Next step was assembling a crew. My first call was to a good friend Wayne who had become an avid kayaker. Without hesitation he agreed to kayak next to me during the swim. Next up were my SWAT brothers and, once again, Ryan and Brian answered the call. The crew also included newcomers Kevin Flanagan and Mike Magri with both being SWAT brothers. Team Valentine was formed!

Days prior to the start I opened my email and discovered a message from Donny Wasser, another SWAT brother. His writing style was captivating, and I had always considered him a warrior poet. The heartfelt note read,

> "Once more to the brink brother!
> God bless you, guard you and fill you with might!
> Think of them dying on far off fields of rock and sand,
> Ponder their valor and sacrifice,
> Say ye your thanks in action!
> With you in spirit, Thanks for your inspiration."

I later had part of this inscribed on a bracelet I wear that includes emergency contact information should I ever be found unconscious on the side of the road during ridiculously long training runs.

On August 28th at 4 pm, we all gathered near the boat launch at Fort Niagara preparing for the start of the swim. The forecast was favorable, and I wanted to start at 5 pm to hopefully take advantage of smooth waters. Most nights the lake calms as the sun sets. Another SWAT brother, Mike Diehl, who I held in very high esteem, made a surprise appearance and was going to kayak next to me for the first three miles. My childhood friend and best man at my wedding, Jim Hildreth, arranged for the Niagara County Sheriff's Department Marine Unit to escort us to Canadian waters.

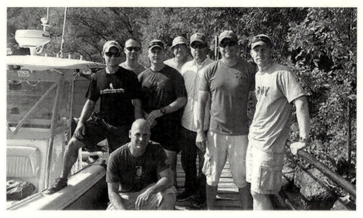

Prior to the start of Swimming for the Seals- Mike Magri, Kevin Flanagan, Mike Diehl, Wayne Burchfield, Jason Aymerich, Brian Sexstone and Ryan Hickey

The deputies were quite a bit older than me, and I could tell they thought I was crazy. Kevin was loading cans of Genesee Light beer into the built-in boat cooler when the deputies intervened. They strongly suggested against taking beer because it was against the law in Canada due to the type of boat we were using. Kevin looked to me for advice and I told him to remove them while waiting for the deputies to walk away. I then whispered to keep half of them in there for the post swim celebration.

After well wishes and hugs from my crew and at exactly 5 pm, I jumped into the lake at the mouth of the Niagara River wearing only a sleeveless wetsuit and swim goggles. Wayne and Mike were next to me in their kayaks. I swam the first three miles like Michael Phelps. This wasn't because of my skills but due to the strong current. The Niagara River dumps super-fast moving water into Lake Ontario after it travels over the Niagara Falls. I was also taking advantage of southerly winds at the time until mile five when the winds switched to the north and the lake turned rough. As the sun began to set, my main goal was to make it to sunrise knowing I would only have nine hours of swimming left. At mile 15 it felt like there were shards of glass in my shoulders every time I rotated them for a swim stroke. I am sure it was from the accumulated lactic acid. The lake continued to churn while the demons questioned if I could make it another 17 miles.

I fully expected what came next. Based on my prior experience at the Beast of Burden, I knew when you dedicate a race or event to a fallen Navy SEAL, they are going to send you some "love." By love I mean adverse conditions to test your fortitude. I began hitting two-foot waves and a strong head-on current. I swam for 30 minutes and only went a quarter mile. I should have gone nearly a mile during that length of time. Kevin later confided that he felt so bad for me a single tear rolled down his face. I remember gritting my teeth while saying, *Thanks Tommy V*, to myself. I was once again squarely at the "crossroads" and had two choices: buckle down and plow ahead or give in a little and ease up. The latter involves first giving up an inch, then a foot, then a mile and ultimately failure. I thought a lot about Tommy, his wife Christina, and Wemo. It took me several hours to swim out of that patch of water and I was proud I had passed the test.

It didn't last long because soon I swam into water that was downright freezing. My hands and feet started to go numb. I swam to Wayne's kayak for some Gatorade and could barely get it in my mouth because I was trembling so badly. I knew hypothermia was settling in, but I also realized the only way to get warm was to swim faster. In addition to that, I had contracted some type of virus. I'm assuming the illness came from all the lake water I had inadvertently drank and needed to immediately remove my wetsuit or it would be full of diarrhea. At this point my lips were purple and my body was shaking uncontrollably. My skin had gone from tan to pale white. While taking it off, I glanced up and saw Mike Magri staring at me. This was his first time seeing me suffer and his eyes had the look of both sadness and deep concern. I knew he felt sorry for me, and I was pissed at him for it. It made me realize just how bad I was feeling. I again thanked Tommy V for the challenge, but I didn't mean it because the thread I was hanging by was about to snap. That was the last of wearing the wetsuit and I went for about two miles until swimming into "warmer" waters. The diarrhea continued for the rest of the swim, and I now had the added concern of becoming dehydrated. I fought hard to make it to sunrise.

That was the first time I had ever seen the moon fully move through the sky. It initially appeared on my right shoulder and eventually disappeared over my left one. The sun rose and the nine hours ahead seemed like an eternity but now I was making good time. That was until the last seven miles. I hit all of the above challenges: strong currents and rough freezing water. It was demoralizing to swim hard while making little progress. In addition to that, hypothermia had set in again and my facial hair had worn a hole through the skin on my left shoulder from breathing exclusively on that side. My mantra became, "swim your way out of this, that's the only way." There would be no more "resting" strokes (sidestroke or breaststroke). I only used the front crawl (freestyle) for the next seven hours. The crew was keeping Christina informed the entire time and passing on her well wishes to me. The one that stuck out was "Great works are performed not through strength but by perseverance." This played in my head like a skipped record and helped to keep me from breaking.

I eventually landed north of a beach near the National Yacht Club exactly 22 hours and 30 minutes from the start. The shoreline consisted of giant seaweed covered rocks and I crawled up on one. I sat there shaking uncontrollably and could feel the vertigo. The boat crew kept yelling for me to stand up for a picture and I knew that was a horrible idea. Like a fool I obliged, well for a second that is. I quickly fell back into the water while pinning my ankle between the rocks causing my body and head to become submerged. I struggled hard to free myself while thinking it would be a shame to drown AFTER the swim. It took all of my courage to re-enter the cold water and swim the 100 yards back to the boat. I felt I was near death.

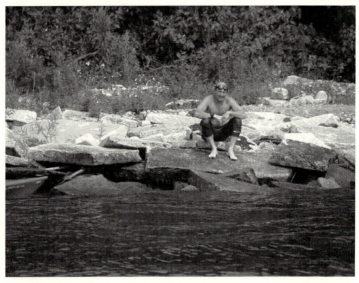

Finally reaching the Canadian shore after 22 ½ hours of swimming

Once back on the boat my brothers put a heavy down camouflage jacket on me while draping an American flag across my back and a SWAT flag across my lap (book cover photo). We motored over to the yacht club and phoned into customs alerting them of our arrival to Canada. That was followed by a giant hamburger and fries at their restaurant, and I instantly began to feel better. The best part was the diarrhea had finally stopped. Immediately after lunch we started our trip back to Fort Niagara.

When we were far enough from land, we began to crack open the cans of Genesee Light to celebrate the adventure. It wasn't long before we ran out of them, and everyone was nursing their last beer. That is when, out of nowhere, a boat sped up behind us with blue and red flashing lights with a booming siren. We attempted to hide our beer like high schoolers who got caught by sheriff deputies drinking in a farm field. I couldn't believe this was happening and felt we were on the verge of receiving some major fines. It was a huge relief when the boat finally pulled alongside us, and we saw it was a US Customs and Border Protection (CBP) vessel. The first person I saw was Jose Garcia who was also on the Colorado elk hunting trip. He and Jason were cousins and I had worked with Jose for many years when he was an Immigration and Naturalization Service special agent. We were very good friends and he now worked for CBP. The next person I saw was CBP Agent Alex Abrue, who I had also worked with back in Rochester. We grabbed their boat and Jose handed me a styrofoam cooler full of iced down Genesee Lights. The good people of Toronto could probably hear our cheers! They told us to follow them and escorted us to the boat launch.

This challenge had been different from the previous running ones. While running I could stop if needed and knew during the hot races it would eventually cool at night. During this I couldn't stop moving or I would drown. There was no escaping perpetual motion. I also couldn't escape the effects of the water. I felt it draining the life from me and there was nowhere to hide from it. This was beyond a doubt the hardest thing I had completed notwithstanding the building of my house. I once again had a new lens to look through and more calluses on my soul. I had experienced true and unadulterated personal greatness. I didn't care if people swam it faster than me, my only concern was that I swam it as fast as I could. That I stayed the course both in training and during the swim while enduring hardship that seemed unfathomable a relatively short time ago. I was only mildly disappointed that I didn't make my time goal. My GPS watch showed I actually swam almost 34 miles. Just because I was born gray, it didn't mean I couldn't be great in my own way. I now felt nothing was impossible if I was determined to accomplish it.

The recovery process took a month and especially concerning were my shoulders. I could barely raise them for a week after the swim and had to feed myself with a fork taped to a butter knife so the food could reach my mouth. I was warned that I may have done some irreversible damage to them but refused to believe that. A regimen of ibuprofen, icing and stretching had them good as new.

A box arrived in the mail, and it contained a custom wooden AIATT longboard. The included note read:

Dear Brett,

I hope you like the small token of my appreciation for your awesome and amazing support of AIATT. Even more than that I want to thank you for honoring Tom and being his friend. I know you swam your butt off and really dug deep both physically and emotionally. It speaks volumes about you and your character. I hope you know how awesome you are!

Always,
Christina

That letter has been stuck to my refrigerator ever since, and the longboard is another item I cherish, just like my team Pierson shirt.

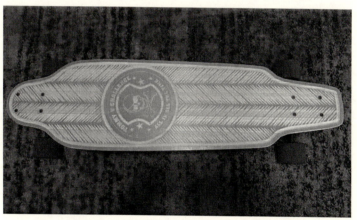

My All In, All The Time Tommy V longboard

My entire crew performed flawlessly and put my needs above theirs. Wayne kayaked next to me the entire time. I am eternally grateful for their brotherhood! One of the goals was to make Tommy proud. Only he knows and many years from now, when I see him, I will personally ask him about the swim.

A month later my mother passed away at the age of 72. She had been diagnosed as having both minor strokes and dementia while in her late fifties and had to be placed in a nursing home. She quickly became nonverbal and failed to recognize me. Early on when we would visit, her eyes would light up when she saw Zachary. He was a spitting image of me in my youth and I believe she thought it was me. Soon afterwards her eyes failed to light at all. Her body was so strong that she lived well past what the doctors had thought was possible. It was hard to visit her because I would always leave crying. I could race until I felt like I was dying but had a hard time summoning the courage to see her frequently. My sister called one day and said mom was in the hospital in Lockport and was near death.

I went to see her, and she was unconscious the entire time. I apologized for not seeing her as often as I should and explained everything good about me came from her, and she was truly the kindest, most unconditional person I had ever known. I also told her it was ok to let go and be with God. She had suffered far too long, and I reassured her Zachary and Gabriel were doing great and missed her. That was the last time I saw her alive. She made it out of the hospital only to die several days later. She never knew of my endeavors, but I know she would have been proud. She always made me feel loved and to her there was nothing gray about me. I once again find myself wiping tears from my face as I write this.

Chapter 10- The Pinnacle

Once again, I received the Dear John letter from Chris Kostman on February 9 regarding my 2016 Badwater 135 race application but this one came with a caveat. It read, "I'm writing to let you know that you are third on the Wait List for the 2016 STYR Labs 135 Ultramarathon. Based on past history, that means you will be accepted into the race at a later date. How soon that will be, I can't predict yet. It could be in a week; it might be in a month or two." Week after week went by without hearing a word. After three months I was resigned to the fact that it wasn't going to happen. I tried my hardest to get in meaningful training, but I felt dejected. My runs kept getting shorter and I wasn't fully engaged while doing them. I would go from being pissed off, knowing I deserved to be in the race, to majorly disappointed, wondering what else I could have done during the application process. I wasn't close to being an elite ultra-marathoner, but I knew I could beat over half the people running it.

On May 18th the other shoe dropped, my father died. He had been diagnosed with lung cancer earlier in the year and had smoked since he was 12. My best estimate is he smoked at least three packs of cigarettes a day. Just before his death and after several rounds of radiation, Zachary and I stopped by his house while out on a motorcycle ride. He looked extremely frail, and I was immediately saddened. During our conversation he said he quit smoking because it was killing him, and he repeated this several times. We said our goodbyes, and on the ride home I couldn't stop thinking, *Dad, smoking had already killed you*. That was the last time I saw him alive. He died at night after his first chemotherapy session. The man I admired most in the world was gone.

Out of nowhere on June 4th I received an email saying I had been selected for the race. It was bittersweet because my father's death was still very raw plus I only had six weeks to plan and train for the race. I wasn't going to say no but I had two choices -- go down to the race, play it safe and finish within the allotted 48 hour time limit. Or, go with a giant chip on my shoulder and try to crush it, because I felt I should have been in the race from the get go. I chose the latter because I wanted to prove a point. I crunched the numbers and decided my goal was to finish in under 34 hours and I immediately began to ramp up my training. Most of my runs had me wearing heavy sweatpants, winter jacket, knit hat and gloves. I knew I needed to get used to being hot, really hot, so I also bought an infrared sauna. I would sit in it for an hour after my runs at a temperature of 140°. I would spend that time stretching and eating.

My longest training run was to be 25 miles on July 4th weekend. I was nearing my house on mile 20 to drink some Gatorade I had stashed in my mailbox, when I saw a local farmer baling hay all by himself. His name was Mr. Waterstreet, and although I had never personally met him, he would always give me a smile and a wave whenever I ran past him while he was out on his tractor.

On this day, he would hop off his tractor after the baler spit out a few bales, stack them and then jump back on his tractor. I'm guessing he was in his mid-70s. With the sun scorching down, I sprinted home and got out of my winter clothes while grabbing a pair of work clothes. He looked at me like I was in a cartoon as I ran through the field and hopped up on his hay wagon. When we finished the field, he thanked me with a firm handshake from his leathered hand and even offered to pay me. It was worth missing those final five miles to help a man that was truly the fabric of rural America.

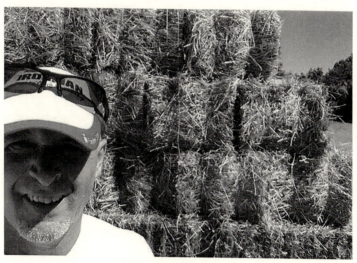

Baling hay with Mr. Waterstreet

My next task was to assemble a crew for the race. Longtime friend Wayne was again the first call and then SWAT brothers Ryan Hickey, Eric Alexander and Kevin

Flanagan agreed to go, all on short notice. Each had helped me during previous challenges, and they had seen me at both my best and worst. They were also the guys I would never want to let down and knew they would do everything humanly possible to help me finish. I couldn't thank them enough for sacrificing their vacation time as well as family time to help me. Ryan would serve as crew chief. They all came fully prepared physically and knew the vast number of racing rules front to back.

Many things happen in threes and the first was when we landed in Las Vegas and discovered my checked bag got lost. Although I had most of my race essential items in my carry-on bag, I needed things in that suitcase. Kevin eventually found it and the crisis was averted. Next was the rental car. I had reserved and paid for a minivan a month prior but was matter-of-factly told they were all out of them. Kevin knew I was coming unglued with the service rep and played the Seinfeld "rental reservation" episode on his phone to lighten the mood. I had to accept a smaller crossover but, before getting into it, we scoured the giant parking garage for a minivan that we could "acquire." We had just about given up when a family returned a white one which was the perfect color for desert racing. Kevin went over to the return guys and a couple minutes later said we had the van. We just had to wait an hour for it to be prepped. The third thing didn't happen until later the next day.

Because of the short notice, all the prime hotels were booked so I settled on the Saddle West Hotel Casino RV Park in Pahrump, NV which was about an hour from race headquarters. As we pulled in, the marquee read "Home of Winning and Feasting" and this became our team motto. It was 110 degrees when we all went for a 3 ½ mile test run. Halfway through my throat was so dry it hurt, and I began wondering what the hell I got myself into.

The following day, Sunday, we went to Death Valley for the pre-race check in and a mandatory meeting. We then ventured out to Badwater Basin, 282 feet below sea level, where the race would start at night. When we got out of the van it was 122 degrees with 28 mile per hour winds. It felt like being behind a fired-up jet turbine. Although my skin felt like it was melting, the heat felt mysteriously good. We all glanced at each other with that, "WTF, we are going to die" look. Things suddenly became very real.

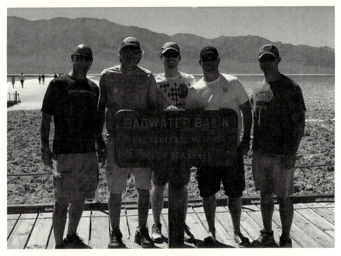

The Badwater Crew- Me, Wayne, Ryan, Eric, and Kevin

There were three starting waves- 8:00 pm, 9:30 pm and 11:00 pm. The elite racers were the last to go and I was in the middle wave. Just prior to starting they played the national anthem and I remembered how proud I was to be an American. While giving last minute hugs to the crew, I told each of them nobody in this wave beats us. A "rule" of ultra-racing is that you should never feel like you are racing because of the vast distance and duration of the race. It's like the other rule that you should never do an Ironman distance triathlon in your first year. Again, who makes these rules up? I know, the guys and gals that have never truly raced an ultra or never did an Ironman in their first year. One should never be fearful of making their own rules or to break existing ones. While I talked about the other runners, I also knew I would be competing against the living, breathing course just like my previous races. Death Valley's job was to break me, and my job was not to be broken. The gun went off and many of the runners got out ahead of me. I let them go because I had 135 miles to catch them. It was still hot as hell with high winds, and I could see sand blowing past my headlamp.

I was running well, and my first marathon split was a respectable 4 hours and 24 minutes. I was holding my own and hit mile 42 at 5:15 am which marked three special occasions. The elite runners began passing me and I wished I had their genes. I then quickly remembered what Wemo had told a fellow SWAT brother when he said he wished he had better reflexes. "Learn to screw with the dick you got, not the one you wish you had." Or in other words, work with what God gave you. Since I was the consummate gray man, I knew I needed to train my mind just as hard, if not harder, than my body. At this time I was also able to have a pacer run with me. Ryan, Kevin, and Eric would take turns running four miles with me and radio ahead to the van via a walkie talkie with what supplies I needed. I was eating and drinking every two miles and it switched between Gatorade, water, and GU chomps (four little chewy squares), and occasionally Drip Drop. At each feeding I would also take two Endurolyte capsules (giant horse pills that contain sodium and other elements). The third thing was that this marked the start of the first climb, a 17-mile, 5000 feet ascent to Towne Pass Summit. This mountain went on forever! We eventually hit the top and then got back to running like we stole something on the steep nine-mile descent. Most racers were pounding the downhill, but I held back a little because I still had the bulk of the race ahead of me. Plus running hard downhill shreds your quads and wreaks havoc on the knees. Just before hitting the next valley that took us to our second climb, I decided to change socks and shoes because I could feel a giant blister forming on my left heel. Many people who know me have heard me jokingly say, when I'm suffering the most during a race, I wish a plane would drop from the sky and land on me to take me out of my misery. I was sitting in a chair changing when I looked up and saw an F-16 fighter jet 200 feet overhead followed by a crack that hurt my ears. Maverick just buzzed our van and Wayne thought a semi-truck had hit it. Everyone flinched and ducked for cover. No more wishing planes dropping from the sky!

It was around noon when we crossed Panamint Valley and I could feel the soles of my shoes getting sticky as they melted from the hot pavement and my feet felt like they were on fire. I touched my dark colored shoes and the heat hurt my fingers. Now when I would pass our van, the guys would wand me down with a pump type weed killer sprayer filled with ice and water. The problem was the water felt warm to me because the hot air would heat the cold water before reaching me. I kept telling them to put ice in it and they would just laugh and say, "There is you jackass." It was that hot and getting hotter!

Our next climb came quickly, and it was a 17-mile, 3500 feet ascent past Father Crowley Point to Darwin. There wasn't a straight portion to this road, it just kept turning. The demoralizing thing was I was certain the summit was just around the corner only to find that the mountain got higher. It was at mile 70 when I went to chew on some GU Chomps, and I saw stars. All the sugar had made my teeth sensitive, and it felt like someone was drilling into them when I bit down on something that contained sugar. All my solid race food contained sugar and I wasn't sure how I was going to make the next 65 miles on liquids. I was nervous and more importantly tired. Because of the time change I didn't sleep well at all in the two nights leading up to the race. I had weaned myself off of coffee two weeks prior so that when I took caffeine in it would really kick start me. I started drinking flat Coke prior to crossing Pananmint Valley but was still tired and had to run through another night. I was nervous because now I could barely keep my eyes open.

When I finally reached Father Crowley Point, tired, sore, and hot, Ryan looked over at me stone-faced and said, "This Father Crowley guy must have been a real jerk." The climb had crushed me. I read a veteran racer say it's when you are climbing to Father Crowley, baking in the sun, you wonder why the hell you are doing this. I didn't wonder why but I was in a bad way. With every step I was wishing for the sun to go down. Somewhere along the climb, I talked to another racer and asked him what time he was hoping to finish in. He said he just wanted to finish, and this wasn't a race where you care about time. He had a right to his own opinion, and I respected it. He asked me about mine and I answered 34 hours. He looked at his watch and I saw him doing the math in his head. He then quipped, "You might want to think about adjusting that upwards four or five hours." I angrily thought to myself, *How about I adjust your face upwards four or five hours*?

He didn't know I was a better second half racer in ultras. It didn't mean I got faster; I just didn't slow down as much as most others do. I wanted to tell him about that "rule" when you do your long training runs and you should take it easy because it's all about spending time on your feet. And how I called bullshit on that sometime ago. If I go out on a 25-mile run, my goal would be to make each mile faster than the last, even if it's just seconds. I wanted to tell how this teaches my body to push harder the more tired I get, the opposite of what is supposed to happen. It's pure and simple brainwashing. I bit my tongue and wished the guy good luck while running from him.

I completed the first 100 miles in just under 24 hours and knew I had 10 more hours to go. It felt good to shed my shirt and hat after the sun had disappeared, but this was when the paradox hit me. It seemed impossible to go on another 10 hours, but I knew I had no choice in the matter. I was at rock bottom and the only way out was to put one foot in front of the other. Wayne later confided in me that he had never seen me like that, and this is the guy who crewed me on both the 22 ½ hour lake crossing and my 29-hour double Ironman. I was living on Gatorade, flat Coke, and Drip Drop. The guys tried to get me to eat solid foods, but I couldn't. The other shoe dropped when I threw up the Endurolytes before they even hit my stomach. I couldn't take another one for the rest of the race. I was actually relieved that I was at rock bottom because the elevator to hell had finally stopped or so I thought. I then started seeing flashes of light followed by extreme darkness. I thought it was a car coming up behind us and I kept looking back but nothing was there. We hadn't seen another racer for hours and dropped every runner I had been sparring with. We had the desert to ourselves. The guys kept looking over at me, but I really couldn't make out their faces. Great, I was losing my vision for some reason. I could see but just barely and to make matters worse I began losing my coordination and was running like a drunk person. I felt myself bumping into the guys and this is when my mother visited me. I could barely see her face, but I could tell her eyes were watering. No mother likes to see their child suffer. I started all of this madness after she had dementia and I don't think she understood what I was doing. She told me it was okay to stop, and I said I couldn't. She did her best to smile and then she was gone. Our exchange saddened me deeply, but I loved feeling her presence.

I could see the lights of Lone Pine in the distance, 22 miles to be exact, but they never got closer. This was the last stop before I tackled Mt. Whitney, the highest point in the contiguous United States. I could slowly feel the course stealing my soul and I got pissed. I was moving on pure willpower and the only emotion I could conjure was rage. I kept telling the course in my head, *Fuck you! I'm not breaking today!* I was at the crossroads and the course had put many demons in my body. They were manifesting themselves as broken feet, loosened toenails, seized calves, throbbing knees and a heavy heart. They got into my head and yelled for me to stop in an attempt to steal my will to carry on. I kept getting more pissed off at them and knew I needed to draw a line in the sand. The line marked how much suffering I could endure. I then needed to step one foot over it. I also knew the demons were going to come at me hard. I was going to take my fair shares of blows but it's all about bracing and holding my ground. When they hit me, I gave them a piss-off-that-wasn't-so-bad smile and dragged a little more of my body over the line. Little by little, I fully crossed that line, and the extreme suffering became my new normal and slightly more bearable. Instead of squarely facing the fire down, I was in the middle of it. It wasn't about rainbows and butterflies but rather controlled rage and pain. It was both mentally and physically taxing to stay on the other side of that line, but I had experienced it during many hours of hard meaningful training. I try to get to this point EVERYTIME I go on a training run. Sometimes it's only for a few fleeting seconds and other times it might be for hours. I was once again standing in the middle of that giant flame and enduring its rath.

Every foot strike felt like the bones in my feet were breaking. It seriously made my eyes water and that's when the Joshua and cactus trees started to magically turn into wolves and sticks into snakes. It was hard to distinguish what was real and what was imagined. I would flinch here and there when they would jump towards me and then I almost stepped on a real snake! The guys said it looked poisonous because it had a triangular head and also looked mad. I would be mad too if I had to live in this God forsaken place.

There were a few times I had to sit because I felt as if I was going to die if I took another step. Then it was back on my feet and across that line again. This is when I saw red lights on Mt. Whitney. They were racer support cars but never seemed to move and that's because the 13-mile ascent to the portal sucked the life out of already fatigued racers. I ran into Lone Pine and began the final leg of the race. The portal road contains 5000 feet of elevation over roughly 11 miles, and I have never been on a road that steep. There were too many switchbacks to count and all the cars descending the mountain road smelled of burning brakes.

Years earlier I had taken over the role of lead PT instructor at the police academy following in the footsteps of the great Todd Baxter. During physical training sessions in the academy, I would often ask the recruits to be "great" during workouts. As we took off up the road,

I remembered thinking that I could be great for this last portion of the race regardless of the shape I was in. It is not morally fair to ask, expect or demand greatness from others and not attempt it yourself. Most runners take six hours to complete this portion, but I had allotted four. The real goal was no stopping whatsoever. I was switching between power walking and running and was completely redlined waiting for the wheels to come off while fighting the urge to rest, if just for a second. This was when my father visited. "How you doing, Pretty boy?" I told him I've been better but holding my own. He replied, "Yes, you are." and then he was gone. I had hoped he was proud.

I broke my promise not to stop because I had to urinate. The sun had risen already, and Ryan was next to me relieving himself when he asked, "Guess who we are peeing in front of?" I answered, "The nun?" To which I received a, "Yes sir!" A female racer we would see now and then had a nun on her crew. At one point she asked my guys to take the nun to her van because she couldn't keep up with her. The guys obliged but the nun was so exhausted and incoherent that she forgot what van was hers. This resulted in my crew riding around with her for a little longer than expected. I'm pretty sure that brings good karma. I looked over and there she was about 20 feet away. It was then back to slaying Mt. Whitney and now I passed a nice German runner. He had been way ahead of me at the start of the climb, and I could tell the mountain had broken him. Kevin, Eric, and Wayne were out of the van at a switch back to cheer me on and, when I passed them, they asked why I was giving them double middle fingers. I didn't even realize I was doing it, but it was for the demons, not my brothers.

My hamstrings and calves were twinging and on fire and I could barely catch my breath. Kevin began walking with me and blurted out, "I'm guessing you have about 2000 steps left before you finish." I would have thrown him off the mountain if I had the strength. I didn't have 20 steps left in me and, after he explained the math, it was more like 4000 steps. This is when I truly began to live in the second because a minute was just too damn long. I developed the following saying over hundreds of hours of training -- "In order to accomplish the seemingly unobtainable goal, you have to do work at it until you feel as though you cannot hold on a second longer. It is in the ensuing seconds, then minutes, then hours and maybe days, when you persevere, that you truly know what it is like to be invincible." This looped in my head. Little by little I was stealing the course's soul while becoming invincible. Ryan looked over at me during the ascent and once again with his stone-face asked, "Why the hell couldn't this be Badwater125?"

The more I climbed the more evil the mountain looked. The crew decided I would run the last half mile by myself, and I knew when they handed me the American flag the race was almost over. I mustered what little energy I had left to cross the finish line running, and like that, it was over in 34 hours and 22 minutes. I carried the flag because I'm damn proud to be an American and this was an international field of racers.

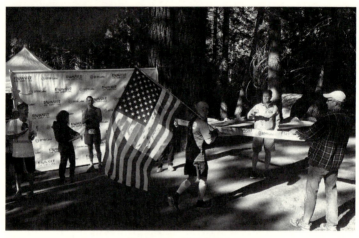

Badwater 135 finish

After a couple pictures and receiving my finisher belt buckle, we hit up the McDonalds at the base of the mountain. I'm guessing I burned roughly 30,000 calories and only took in 7000. I nearly had one of everything on the breakfast menu. Two days after the race I was still down 11 pounds and didn't recognize my own body. I slept like the dead on the three-hour ride back to the hotel and didn't even wake up during driver changes. Before drifting off, I did see many of the runners I had passed still out on the course, and I felt extremely sorry for them. The desert was heating up again fast.

My crew are not just friends, they are brothers! Wayne drove the van the entire time except for a mile in which he accompanied me up Mt. Whitney. Kevin,

Ryan, and Eric each ran 31 miles with me, and everyone stayed awake during the race. Oh, the third omen. The day before the race, Ryan broke a toe in a freak accident. He hobbled the entire day and before the race he taped it to his other toe to immobilize it. Thirty-one miles on a broken toe and not one complaint. The guys remained positive the entire time and suffered greatly at my expense. I hope one day to repay the favor and I certainly would not have finished without them. I love them as brothers, plain and simple!

This was by far the hardest physical thing I had ever done. I tend to oversimplify things in my head and had an idea as to how difficult it would be. It ended up being three times as difficult as I had originally thought. I left part of my soul out there but replaced it with course's soul. I finished 29th out of 97 racers and 22 minutes over my time goal. I'm still mad at myself for sitting those times during the race but I have no real regrets. At the risk of jinxing myself, it cemented my personal belief that I can't be broken if I am fully committed to the task at hand. Was I still gray? Absolutely! Did I experience personal greatness during my adventure through Death Valley? Absolutely!

Chapter 11- A Hard Lesson Learned

2017 found me doing several races to include the Winter Beast of Burden 100 miler. My rationale for doing it was I had never enjoyed running in the cold and thought this would add an additional challenge. Be careful what you wish for comes to mind when I look back at that race. At one point I was convinced I was freezing to death. It had snowed for most of the race and there was a strong west wind that pounded me on every return trip to Lockport from Middleport.

I pretty much had the same SWAT brothers as pacers. Kevin Flanagan and my son Gabriel crewed me the entire time with Kevin pacing me on the final leg. New to my team was friend Bob Lonsberry and his son Lee. Several police recruits ran the last three miles with me, as did Todd. He was still recovering from prostate cancer but that did not stop him. Once again, I raised money for the VOC, and this became Running for the Vets II.

At times I am saddened when a race ends but was relieved when this one was over. I had shivered for the last half of the race and was saved when Scott Peters literally gave me the coat off his back while he was pacing me with Pete Brunett. I often think back to that race while lacing up my shoes for outdoor runs during winter storms and think, *I've been here before and survived, so let's go!*

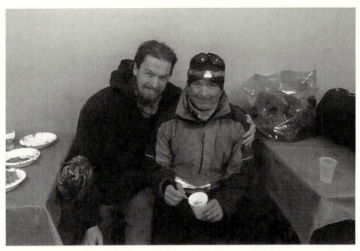

The Winter Beast of Burden at mile 88 ½ with my son Gabriel

In May I ran the Mind the Ducks ultra-marathon, a 12-hour race around a 1.01 mile paved trail at North Ponds Park in Webster, NY. I was doing great right up to the six hour mark with 38 miles completed. In fact I was staying with the leaders, one of whom was a finisher of the famed Barkley Marathons. Upon leaving the bathroom after a quick pit stop, and out of nowhere, I felt a shooting pain in my left knee. I tried to run it off but after limping around the course for two miles, I quit the race. I packed up my things and abruptly left. I didn't try to work it out like I had done at the Double Anvil race.

It was difficult for me to process "why" I quit. I had persevered during the run portion of my Double Anvil triathlon race with a sore knee for over 50 miles. I continued swimming for a half a day when my shoulders were literally shredded to pieces. I ran through the fiery pit of hell at Badwater 135 while working through heat exhaustion, sleep deprivation and crippling digestive issues. Yet on this day, I casually walked off the course in defeat. I looked back at my training logs and discovered I put in enough physical run training. The answer then became apparent. I failed to train my mind and soul like I had before.

I was coming off of my Badwater 135 finish which was the last item on my bucket list. It truly was the pinnacle, and I was very content with my recent accomplishment. My ego made me think, *It's only a 12 hour race,* and I woefully underestimated it. I tried to break myself here and there during training but not like before. I took for granted that my mental toughness was indelibly etched into me like a tattoo. I had failed to develop that, "The only way I'm leaving this race is by finishing or die trying" mentality. I learned the harsh lesson that past successes are good teachers but they by no means guarantee future successes. I had temporarily abandoned what brought me to discover personal greatness in the first place, an indestructible mindset forged through very mindful training.

I spent well over a decade preaching to police recruits about never quitting but there I was a quitter and worst of all, a hypocrite. That decision tormented me every single day for the following year and frequently haunts me to this day. Every time I drove by the course during that first year, I felt its smug smirk, with its middle finger fully extended telling me, "I owned your punk ass." I was pissed but again, the loser never gets to dictate how the victor celebrates. I needed payback. I needed redemption. Most of all, I needed peace of mind.

The following year I returned to the Mind the Ducks, and with fists cocked full of bad intentions, looked for revenge. I trained hard, not quite like my life depended on it hard because of intense work obligations, but very meaningful training. I returned to trying to break myself during every training run. I developed those new calluses on my soul until it was bulletproof. I thought back to past challenges I had conquered and used them as springboards during training. My mantra during runs was "try or die" meaning those were the only two options on race day. As the race grew closer, I felt like the old me, the guy that was subdued but confident in his abilities. Deep down I knew I was willing to risk much should the need arise. I felt a certain level of anxiousness but no fear, even though I knew the course had it out for me.

I ran that race with much confidence mixed with a little rage. Some of it was directed at the course but most was pointed back at me because I was the one who decided to walk off it last year. There were the normal discomforts like sore feet, stinging toenails, and swelling blisters but not one could break through to my armored soul. There was one point when the proverbial thread was stretched very thin but this year it was made of Kevlar. I had turned my ankle when running on the edge of the paved trail while passing several other runners. It was borderline painful for several miles but there was no way in hell I was going to let it defeat me. Eventually it began to feel better and at best it became a mild inconvenience.

I finished my last lap just before the 12 hours was up and completed 66.8 miles. I felt a smile come across my face knowing that I had "beat" the course. I was hoping this would get the monkey off my back that had been torturing me for the past year. My efforts had me winning the Male Veteran Award which I call the old man division for racers over 50 years of age. I slept well that night.

Chapter 12- Farther Yet

Both the lake swim and Badwater 135 had pushed me to the edge- mentally, physically, and spiritually. After some reflection, I debated if I had really stared down at the pity of failure. The true canyon floor where breaking lives. I began searching for a new challenge and was contemplating 200-mile races out west. That changed when I learned of a pending retirement at my department.

Lt. John Prewasniak, known as Pre to most, was a champion for Special Olympics for as long as I could remember. He helped to organize and raise money through events such as the Law Enforcement Torch Run, Polar Plunge and Cops on Tops. Pre was always recruiting officers for these events, and you could sense his passion. He's a man who always wore a smile and shied away from recognition.

I racked my brain trying to think how I could return a small part of the dedication he had shown for Special Olympics for so many years. I thought of it as my retirement gift to him. After coming up empty for several days, I woke up in the middle of the night with the answer. I would run 48 hours straight to raise awareness and money for Special Olympics New York. I ran the idea by him during his final work days and his ear-to-ear smile said it all. He also appeared to be incredibly surprised. It goes to show that one never truly knows how much their passion and deeds impact others. He had no idea of my great admiration for him. I was silently inspired by his deep commitment and, more importantly, tireless efforts. Thank you, Pre!

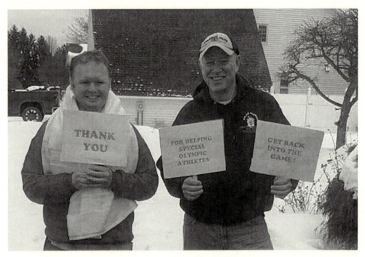

Special Olympic athlete Jacob Babcock and
Lt. John "Pre" Prewasniak

He told me he would introduce me to the Special Olympics fundraising folks at his retirement party and it was there where I met Kelley Ligozio and Luke Folts. I enthusiastically ran the idea by them, and they were immediately sold with one caveat. Luke suggested I run for 50 hours to coincide with the 50th anniversary of the national organization in 2018. His exact words were, "What's another 2 hours?" I spontaneously thought, *a shit ton!* I lied though, and said it would be nothing. We agreed the run would be called "50 for 50 with Brett Sobieraski- Special Olympics New York."

Now I needed to establish a route for the run, and that was the easy part. I chose the canal path due to lack of vehicular traffic and ease of access. The path would also allow me to travel through numerous towns and villages making the resupplying of food and drink easy. I would start at Broderick Park in Buffalo which was a very meaningful place. On October 13, 2017, Officer Craig Lehner of the Buffalo Police Department drowned in the adjacent Niagara River during a SCUBA training exercise. The park served as a makeshift memorial for him. The run would follow the river and eventually turn onto the canal path. I would wind my way through Niagara, Orleans, Monroe, Wayne, Cayuga and hopefully Onondaga counties. I set a goal of running 200 miles during the 50 hours and that would have me ending in Syracuse.

I immediately began training and, once again it revolved around long runs, backup runs, negative splits and attempts to break myself. I tried to make it as brutal as possible knowing I couldn't train my body to run 50 hours however, I could train my brain. I went back to singularly concentrating on the actual run during training. I would visualize running portions of the route during each session. This challenge would be almost 16 hours longer than Badwater and I tried my best to stop reminding myself of that.

On July 13th, the day before my 52nd birthday, I stood at Broderick Park ready to start running at 9 am. My son Zachary hugged me and told me he was proud of me. The thought of that and Officer Lehner made my eyes water for the first mile. I wore a camelback back-pack and carried a credit card. There were no pacers or crew to aid me, but I extended an open invitation for anyone to join in along the way. Hundreds of coworkers, friends and complete strangers either ran with me or cheered me on. Each time they did I would steal a little bit of their souls and add it to mine. Each encounter was another log on the fire, and it would be impossible to tell you of each experience. I will share a few of them with you.

The hot sun had set, and I had made it into Orleans County while feeling depressed and tired. Sergeant Jay Vislay, who taught physical training with me at the police academy, called me and said he was coming out. It was just what I needed. We met at a bridge, and he came bombing down the steep bank with a bike over his shoulder. He had an extremely sore back but that didn't stop him. I was sitting on a bridge footing while eating and drinking when I laid down on it. The cool concrete felt good on my sweaty back. It had been a ridiculously hot day. I didn't want to get back up and felt myself drifting into sleep. I immediately told myself I needed to get up in three seconds and start running. At the end of the countdown, I had sprung to my feet and took off like a bat out of hell. I yelled to a startled Jay to grab my camelback while speeding away. He caught up to me and was still stunned at what had happened. Jay said it looked like I got shocked with a defibrillator. I had gotten my second wind! Jay rode his bike next to me for eight hours and I was sad when he departed. He went on to take over the academy PT program when I retired. Jay also ran and completed the Beast of Burden in 2021. I happily paced him the last 25 miles.

Before entering into Monroe County, Todd, Bob Lonsberry, and Todd's son Zach joined us, which also included friends Kimmy Sawyer and Charlene Fry, who we had picked up several miles ago. Bob was instrumental in my fundraising by having me on his radio show several times and hyping the run to his huge social media following.

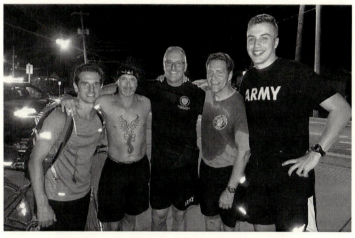

Entering Monroe County with Jay Vislay, Todd Baxter, Bob Lonsberry, and Zach Baxter

Upon approaching the county line I saw revolving red and blue lights and a string of officers from different agencies standing in formation. Todd had arranged for this and was now the Sheriff of Monroe County. I had taught most of these 10 officers in the academy. Recruits who I had at one time asked to be great. Their presence added jet fuel to my veins and the fatigue magically left my body. We began hammering out mile after mile at a blistering pace for the next seven miles.

Todd didn't tell me but as a parting gift he had arranged for Monroe County Sheriff's Office (MCSO) deputies to be at every bridge whenever feasible. My mini goal was to make it to sunrise firmly believing the start of a new day would recharge me. Every time I saw those revolving lights and sworn protectors it was an instant shot of adrenaline. These were my brothers and sisters, and I would never want to let them down. The sun eventually rose and so did my spirits.

When I arrived at Schoen Place in Pittsford it had a carnival type atmosphere. Dozens of people lined the canal and I had been running with Pre and Investigator Erin Rogers, who had taken over Pre's role as department liaison with Special Olympics. MCSO cars lined the street with more of my past recruits greeting me. The day was once again heating up and I stopped to pop a handful of blisters on my feet and toes. My girlfriend Laura also joined in the run. She looked a little concerned because this was her first time seeing me like this.

My last stop in Monroe County was Fairport and SWAT brother Brian had jumped in. Another SWAT brother was supposed to run with me but as luck would have it, the Team got activated. Before I knew it, I was alone during the 10-mile trek to Macedon in Wayne

County. The sun, relentlessly beating down on me, coupled with fatigue and sleep deprivation caused me to become lonely and depressed. The despair I felt was overwhelming as I paused under a bridge to escape the sun's rays. *What are you going to do?* The last 30 hours of running felt like a full week. It was in that moment, with my toes tightly curled over the edge, I found the answer. *You know you're not going to quit, so why are we having this conversation?* I suddenly stopped feeling sorry for myself and got back to running.

Once in Macedon and while running through a trailer park situated on the canal, I was fairly sure I began hallucinating. Running towards me was a pretty lady wearing a sports bra and shorts. I blinked my eyes a few times while wishing this imaginary lady would run with me. She began waving and yelling my name and realized it was no hallucination, it was Tyler MacNeal. I had never met her but knew her husband Steve. We had worked together on my drug task force when he was with the Irondequoit Police Department. He now worked for the Macedon Police Department. We ran for several miles and Steve joined us wearing his uniform. I was a little confused until he reminded me why.

In April of 2017, I was working overtime in uniform at the Rochester Regional Health Half Marathon when I crossed paths with Bob who was running it with his daughter Hannah. He snapped a picture of us and posted it to social media. Todd tweeted that I could probably do the race in uniform...damn you, Todd but thank you!

The next year I found myself running it in full uniform to include a bulletproof vest, fully equipped gun belt and boots.

Speaking of Bob, he now joined me for the second time. He also brought me ice cold Gatorade that never tasted so good. It was like a gift from the heavens. I began to feel exceptionally well considering the circumstances and knew it was because of the company. Other great folks joined in, and I was eventually met by SWAT brother Kevin who was wearing a giant backpack. He had enough supplies for a week.

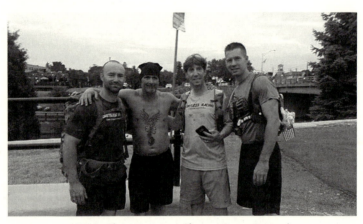

Kevin Flanagan, me, Shawn Gorman, and
Andrew Loughlin in Newark

We ran and ran and ran some more until it got dark. Pre phoned and told us they were going to shut down the road on the canal in Lyons because of fireworks. Next thing I knew we were sprinting two miles to beat the closure. I was exhausted but we made it only to learn that the canal path actually ended. Out of nowhere Sgt. Martin Cozens, a member of the National Guard who was assigned to my narcotics units, appeared, and pointed us to a trail he thought would get us back to the canal while paralleling us in his car. We never did find the canal and ran country roads towards Clyde. I had developed giant bloody rashes on my inner thighs and stopped to apply anti-chafing cream to them. What I failed to realize was I had been wiping my sweaty forehead with my hands. Upon applying the cream, my thighs began stinging and it reminded me of the incident with Gabriel and the alcohol wipes. The problem now was I had nothing to rinse it with and the more I ran the more it hurt to the point of becoming excruciating. Through my winces I could see Pre giving me the same look Mike had given me during the swim. The look of pity. It maddened me just like before because it reminded me of the fragile condition I was in. We soldiered on and it eventually subsided.

At a convenience store in Clyde, Pre and Kevin informed me they were leaving. I didn't say it, but this was a giant blow because I wanted them to stay. One was the man who set me on this course because of his example and the other I had often trusted with my life. I once again slipped into depression as I sat on a curb eating a piece of pizza. I knew I was in a bad way because pizza always makes me happy but not this time. Luke, Erin, and Laura arrived, and I mustered every ounce of strength to get off that curb. I tried to think of positive things but all I felt was pain. My entire being hurt and the demons were throwing haymakers at me. Now I was over the edge and hanging by my fingers. The fall felt imminent until I thought back a few short hours ago when I got mad at Pre for feeling sorry for me. Now I was doing it! *"Hypocrite…hypocrite…hypocrite"* kept looping in my head. It's one of the things I despised, and I was being one.

I made myself run and slowly scorched those demons out of me. I was still on the edge but now standing instead of hanging. The road from Clyde to Port Byron lasted for an eternity. This was where I actually began hallucinating. As we approached a house, I noticed a young child near a swing set and found it odd because it was 2 am. I voiced my concern to Laura and Erin, and they looked hard for the child. They only saw a smaller garbage can next to the swing set and then so did I. An hour later I noticed two horses in a front yard and asked if they wanted to pet them with me. Confused, they kept asking me where and I quietly pointed, so I didn't scare the horses. They hesitantly told me they were bushes, and a look of disappointment came over my face.

Make it to sunrise, once again was my mantra and goal. I tried not to think about the remaining five hours after that; I just wanted to see the sun. We reached Port Bryon just as it crested the horizon and found Luke dead asleep in his car. I chuckled to myself, "What's another two hours?"

The sun changed everything, and I began replacing soreness and tiredness with rage. This course had its way with me all night long and I wanted payback. I quickened my pace to Weedsport. When I got there, I needed to tend to my left foot. I knew a large blister the size of my fist had formed on the front part of my sole. While Luke went to find duct tape, I popped and drained it. This was when June Worden showed up and introduced herself. She was a retired NYS Trooper and was heavily involved in Special Olympics in the central part of the state. She looked at my foot and blurted out, "That's badass!" I knew we were going to get along well.

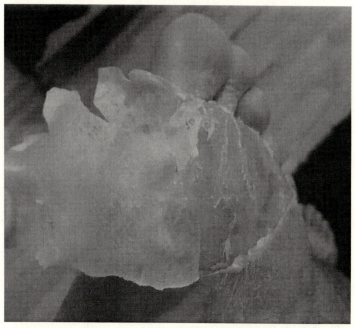

That blister three days after the run

I had less than three hours left and the realization that I wasn't going to make it to Syracuse sank in. June knew the area and arranged for us to end at the trooper barracks in Elbridge, just inside of Onondaga County. After taping up my foot, we headed for the barracks. For a third day the sun beat down on me, but I didn't care, I just wanted to finish. With four miles to go, we needed to park a car and approached a pleasant young lady who was in her yard. She was more than happy to accommodate us, and my partners told her of my journey and then my feet. She was a nurse and offered to look at them. I politely declined knowing we were now racing against the clock to arrive by 11 am.

Before reaching the barracks, I saw Kevin Baxter, Todd's oldest son and he jumped in with us. Then I heard Todd yell my name and he was with his wife Mary. Next, I saw Kayla McKeon. She is a Special Olympic athlete, as well as the first registered lobbyist with Down syndrome, and was holding a flaming Olympic torch. I could feel my eyes welling up. With a trooper car as our escort, Kayla and I held the torch together to the finish. We were received by Kevin Flanagan and his bride Sara, other troopers, and Stacey Bohne Hengsterman and her family. She is the president and CEO of Special Olympics New York. There were also other Special Olympics athletes to include her son. Somehow, she learned of my favorite beer and secretly handed me a can of Genesee.

Instead of drinking it I held it against the back of my neck to cool me.

It was over, 176 miles in 50 hours. After pictures and hugs, we went back to get Laura's car and that nice young lady left a note under the wiper blade. She again offered to bandage my feet for the ride home. She went on to thank me for what I had done, saying she was happy there were people like me in the world. I felt the same way about her.

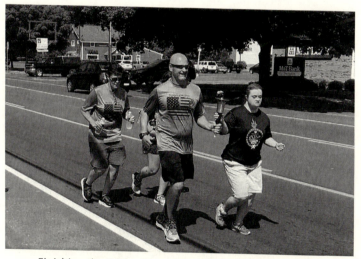

Finishing the 50 for 50 with June Worden, Erin Rogers, and Kayla McKeon

I slept the entire ride home and immediately limped down the stairs of Laura's pool to wash off days of sweat and grime. Once that was done, the uncontrollable shaking started, and I slept on a chaise lounge under a pile of towels in the direct sunlight. Laura was concerned for my wellbeing, but I convinced her this was expected. Physically, it hurt to just breathe that day and my feet were the worst for wear with blisters, dead toenails, and bruised bones. The fact that I wore the same socks and shoes for the entire run didn't help matters. With each subsequent challenge my recovery time was shortened. I was back to running, albeit short and slow, within two weeks.

Mentally, the run pushed me further to the edge than anything prior. Part of me was melancholy that it was over, and the other part was relieved. Relieved I didn't break. Relieved I didn't let my loved ones down. Relieved I didn't let myself down. I had experienced yet another level of suffering and endured it. It's amazing how alive I feel when a part of me feels like it's dying. It's never pretty but there are the most genuine feelings. You can't cover your weaknesses and fears with false bravado when you are completely inside out. I was sad that no angels visited me, but I don't get to choose when they appear, they do.

We surpassed our fundraising goal of $10,000 by over $4,000, while missing my distance goal by 24 miles. It was disappointing and I found myself scheming how I could have run faster. The only thing I would have changed was the first 70 miles when I ran by myself. There were stops at Tops Supermarket, an ice cream stand, a bar for ice water, a hotdog stand and pizza shop.

I admittedly ate an entire medium pizza while running and stole that idea from Dean Karnazes. I also fully realized it was all the folks that helped and/or cheered during the run that fueled me more than any food or Gatorade could. Many sacrificed much so I could succeed, and I am eternally grateful for it.

Chapter 13 - A Grand Run

My friend Bob Lonsberry ran across the Grand Canyon to celebrate his 60th birthday in 2019. The telling of his experience lit a flame inside of me and I soon found myself rather abruptly committing to running across the Grand Canyon and back nonstop. This is commonly referred to as Rim to Rim to Rim. It would be roughly 45 miles with over two miles of elevation gain. Thanks Bob! I set a completion time goal of 12 hours that I knew would be aggressive.

I mainly trained by constantly running up and down several local steep hills with my girlfriend, Laura. This was also mixed in with my typical longer runs followed by shorter ones the next day. My one fault was I did not do a lot of off-road running; however, I did compete in an 18-mile trail race six months earlier. I must admit I never really enjoyed having to constantly look down while running like one has to on trails. This lack of train-ing would come back to mildly haunt me.

I arrived in Arizona on September 15, 2020, and rushed to see the Grand Canyon for the first time. It was absolutely spectacular and the sheer magnitude of it made me feel insignificant. I once again had that in-over-my-head feeling that I had grown accustomed to. The plan was to begin at 5 am the next day and run down the seven mile South Kaibab Trail, seven miles through the canyon floor that is commonly referred to as "the Box," and then seven miles up the North

Kaibab Trail to the north rim. Once there, I would run back down the trail, through the box again, but this time take the 10-mile Bright Angel Trail to return to the south rim.

The next morning I found myself frantically searching for the South Kaibab trailhead in the dark. I was unable to scout this area the day before because the gates were locked and the only way to access it was via a shuttle bus from the main Grand Canyon parking lot. I eventually heard the clicking of hooves on rocks discovering a mule train had made it to the trailhead before I did. The mules are used to pack supplies to the Phantom Ranch which is located on the canyon floor. This slightly delayed my start because I did not want to have to pass them in the dark on the narrow trail. I took the extra time to record a video for social media. My intent was to share parts of my journey with my friends. The video went like this...

"Good morning! I'm coming at you from the south rim of the Grand Canyon getting ready to start my Rim to Rim to Rim run. It will be about 45 miles and I'm repping one of my favorite charities, All In, All The Time. If you get a chance, visit their website. They have some cool gear there and if you have a few dollars in your pocket, you can give them a contribution. They would really appreciate it as would I. COVID has hit them hard with their fundraising. I hope to share a few messages along the way and I'm hoping this takes

12 hours or less. The first message is procrastination. We are a society of kicking that can down the road. We have to stop doing that. There is never a perfect time to start things, there is only THIS time to start things ... now. I was going to plan this for next June and I'm thinking I might not be as trained physically as much as I should be, but why am I going to wait until June? Tomorrow is promised to no one. I will be talking to you soon."

After giving the mules a healthy head start, I began my run while using a headlamp to illuminate the uneven, rocky trail. Part of me was glad that I couldn't see over the edge because I have a healthy fear of heights. I soon discovered that running down this rugged trail was much harder than running down the paved roads back home. I was exerting much more energy dodging and hopping over large rocks. The constant unevenness of the terrain really shocked me, and it wasn't long before I rolled my right ankle by landing on an odd shaped rock. While I was thinking it was much too early in the run for this to happen, it occurred again. My first instinct was to lament about not doing enough trail running in preparation for this adventure, but I quickly reminded myself that wouldn't change a thing right now. Little by little, the discomfort in my ankle faded and I had now caught up to the mule train, as the sun was rising. After a mile or so the riders pulled the mules to the side allowing me to pass.

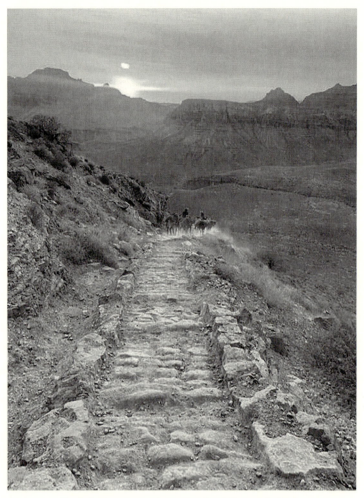

Early in my run as I approached the mule train

I ran for another 20 minutes before catching my first glimpse of the Colorado River. It looked like a post-card, and I stopped momentarily to enjoy the grandeur of it. It helped me to forget the fact that my legs were already feeling a little tired although I was still on the easier downhill portion. I continued on to a twenty foot tunnel carved into a giant stone wall. It was pitch dark and much cooler in the middle of it. Upon exiting, I crossed a narrow suspension bridge over the river and recorded this message ...

"Good morning. I made it down into the canyon floor which is called the box, and I'm on a suspension bridge, which is pretty cool. No doubt God made this place with his hands. It is so impressive down here. What I want to talk about while crossing this bridge is personal greatness. Don't worry about what Mr. and Mrs. Jones are doing. Who cares? Worry about yourself! You have to find your own personal greatness. What does that mean? You have to set goals. It's not just going to come along. So set a goal. It could be physical fitness, it could be secondary education, it could be job related. Set a goal and train for it like it could cost you your life because depending what goal you pick, it could. Personal greatness comes at a cost, comes with sacrifice, toil, uncomfortableness. Find your own personal greatness! Be great! When it comes you will know it. I'll talk to you when I'm on the north rim."

I had finally reached level ground and after a mile or so, I reached the Phantom Ranch. There were nine cabins scattered about along with some larger buildings. I couldn't help but wonder how the heck this place got here, because it resembled a mirage in the middle of the desert. The Phantom Ranch Canteen, a dining hall and small store was open, and I ordered a tall glass of lemonade. It was like a special treat when compared to the lukewarm water in the camelback I wore on my back. I began running again while reminding myself to enjoy the relatively flat trail. The sun began creeping higher in the sky and the box was already heating up when I arrived at the Cottonwood Campground. I stopped to fill my now depleted camelback from a water spigot while trying not to dwell on what came next.

I was now on the North Kaibab Trail and the farther I went, the steeper it got. There were some very narrow portions where I found myself scraping my body against the inside rock face to avoid getting too close to the edge. There was no way of escaping the sun's rays while on this trail. My calves began aching and I wasn't sure if it was from the steep grade or dehydration. I was now alternating between power walking and running because the grade was so steep. I hit switchback after switchback until finally making it to the Supai Tunnel, which was a short cave cut through the rock. I again filled my camelback knowing the last two miles were going to be brutal.

By now I was no longer running, and it took every ounce of willpower not to rest after several steps. I kept telling myself, *Get to the top!* Those last two miles felt like 20, and then all of a sudden, I had reached the trailhead on the north rim. Bob had finished his journey here and I began feeling envious of him. For me it was anti-climactic knowing I had to turn around and relive the hell I had just gone through. I paused for a moment to compose myself while recording this message ...

"Good afternoon or whatever time it is. It has been a while since I checked in and I'm about to head down. I wasn't feeling it for a while so this message is about discomfort. We often mistake discomfort for pain. Those are two entirely different things. When you put your hand on a hot stove that is probably pain but don't get that confused with discomfort. The body can take discomfort for a long, long time. You need to subject yourself to that. Discomfort builds resilience, resilience builds character and character is the foundation of both physical and mental toughness. If you are uncomfortable then accept that as your new normal. Talk to you soon."

I was mad at this portion of the trail for beating me up, so I figured it was my turn for revenge. I knew full well that running hard downhill puts tremendous stress on the knees and shreds the quadriceps, but I didn't care. I tried my best to control the rage I felt inside, and slowed at every narrow switchback to avoid running off the side of the canyon. I continued to run hard on the short straight sections. I would smile now and then while asking the trail, "How does it feel now?" I could feel my breathing become more and more labored, but I didn't try to fight it or reel it back in. My only mission was to run hard until reaching level ground but with that came the consequence of rolling my right ankle for a third time. This one felt different and caused me to wince. I fought the natural instinct to stop and access the damage and continued hard down the trail while willing the sharp pain to go away.

I had finally reached the box and again made a pit stop at the Cottonwood Campground. I immediately noticed it was much hotter now. The sun had heated up the nearly vertical narrow canyon walls and it felt like being in an oven. I knew the temperature was over 100 degrees and the sun scorched my back while the stone wall cooked my left side. There was no way of escaping it because there was no shade. I continued to run, and my only thought was to make it to the Phantom Ranch. I continually drank from the tube of my camelback but still felt dehydrated. My calves were as hard as rocks and my hamstrings began to involuntarily twitch as if they were about to seize up. Before long, the camelback was empty, and I resorted to drinking from a water bottle I carried in case of an emergency. I felt like this constituted one. This adventure was different from my previous ones because it was so desolate. There was no cellular reception and help was never just around the corner. At a bare minimum, it was many hours away. I tried to banish those thoughts and knew the faster I reached the ranch, the better off I would be.

When I finally arrived, I ordered another lemonade but asked for extra ice in it. After gulping it down I placed several of the ice cubes under my hat to cool me. I swear I heard the sizzle of bacon in a skillet as the melting water ran down my back. I put the rest of the ice in my camelback because the thought of drinking warm water made me want to vomit. After filling it the rest of the way with water, I drank directly from the spigot until I felt like my stomach was going to burst. As I began to move, my left calf balled up and it stopped me in my tracks. Luckily, I was next to a picnic table and was able to sit down as opposed to falling down. While trying to massage it away, a little demon crept into my head and asked why the hell am I doing this. The demons always ask questions like that when I'm struggling. A halfhearted smile come across my face while thinking, *Because I can.* With that, I was back on my feet and running again.

It wasn't long until I reached another suspension bridge that crossed the Colorado River, and I recorded this message …

"Checking in. I just made it through the box of the canyon and crossing another suspension bridge. I'm headed towards the Bright Angel Trail, so I have about nine miles left and 5000 feet of elevation. It's a good time to talk about demons. Those voices in your head. Those aches you have, that discomfort, blisters on your feet, loose toenails, sore tight calves, discomfort in your hips. Those are demons! Their job is to get in your head and make you slow down; make you doubt yourself or what you are doing. Your job is not to listen. If they get so loud that you can't help but listen, then flip them off. Smile back at them. The whole goal is to become your demon's demon. Have your demons check under their beds looking for you at night. You be their boogeyman, so they become afraid to show their faces. Nine miles

left and about eight hours into it. The Grand Canyon (as I pan my camera 360 degrees), is not going to be so grand when I get done with it."

I was turned inside out and experiencing every bit of what I said.

The beginning of my ascent surprised me because the first mile was almost all sand, which made running all the more difficult. The trail wasn't initially steep, and I took advantage of this by running hard. I made it to the river Resthouse after 1.5 miles however, there would be no resting here because there was no water spigot. I felt the next three miles sucking the life out of me, and I had drunk the last of my water just before reaching Indian Garden. It was still extremely hot out and the lukewarm water did little to cool me when I ran it over my head. There was a man in his 50s sitting on a shaded bench and asked me where I had hiked from. His eyes grew large when I told him of my journey, and he said he didn't know it was possible to cover that much ground in that amount of time. I took that as a huge compliment but then he ruined it by telling me the trail begins to get really steep after this. He started up the trail while I filled my camelback.

I was surprised at how long it took me to finally catch up with him. He was walking while use trekking poles and making great time. I jokingly asked him if I could borrow them. He went on to tell me that he hikes this trail once a week. I responded that I felt like I never wanted to run it again. As I got out in front of him,

I thought he sure wasn't lying about it getting steeper. My breathing had become more labored, and my calves were once again about to seize up. I willed them not to and switched off between walking and running. The switchbacks became more prevalent which means the grade was becoming steeper. I fought the urge to sit on the various rocks that were of seat height. As I rounded a corner, I saw a young man sitting on such a rock hunched over. I asked him if he was ok, and he barely lifted his head to talk to me. He said he had been vomiting and felt weak. He was wearing jeans and sneakers and I could tell he was in over his head. He went on to say he didn't think it would be that hard to go down three or four miles. I could tell that he was in the early stages of heat exhaustion and asked if he had water. He simply nodded his head no. I gave him my emergency bottle while checking my cellphone for a signal and there was none. I asked if I could see his cellphone and he explained the battery had died. He handed it to me and luckily it was the same brand as mine. I retrieved my small battery charging pack and cable from my camelback and plugged it into his phone. I knew the next stop was less than a half mile away and encouraged him to get on his feet. He flat out refused, and I told him I would try to call for help once I got there. As I walked away from him, I remember thinking that he looked exactly the way I felt.

I reached the Three Mile Resthouse and still did not have reception on my phone. I worried for him while filling my camelback and wasn't sure what to do. I looked over my shoulder and there was the man with the trekking poles. He immediately thanked me for giving the young man my battery pack and water bottle. I explained I didn't have cellular service and he told me my phone carrier doesn't work well in the canyon but his did. He said he had already called the park rangers. As we parted ways, the gentleman told me I was a good man and that lifted my spirits.

It was back to grinding out the last three miles and the trail got steeper with each step. The demons wanted me to stop and rest but I fought that urge with every stride. When I felt I couldn't resist any longer, I would start running to remind myself that walking wasn't that bad. *Don't stop! Don't stop!* was on loop in my head. As I rounded a switchback, I came upon two young women who were blocking the trail. Both of them were hunched over with their hands on their knees gasping for air. This caused me to stop and immediately both of my calves locked up. One of the ladies said, "We are struggling." I asked if she had a cellphone. She said they both did, and I told them they may have to call 911 if they can't make it out. I was barely able to stand because of my calves and kindly told them I needed to get by. They moved to the side so I could shuffle past them. The more I walked, the more my calves unlocked, and I couldn't help but think how many people get beat up by the Grand Canyon on a daily basis.

I realized that stopping to rest would be detrimental to me finishing. Everything below my waist ached and I knew it would only get worse if I stopped moving. My adventure started to feel like a death march, but I had been to this place of suffering before. I suddenly looked up and saw several sheep on the path and a man on the other side looking at them. As I walked past the sheep, they moved down the steep rocks and I apologized to the man for spooking them. I explained that I couldn't stop for fear of my legs seizing up. He was in his mid-twenties and wearing only shorts and high-top sneakers. He told me his name was Tim and explained he started casually running down the trail and before he knew it, he was about one mile into it. *Damn,* I thought, hoping I had less than a mile to go. He began walking with me and did most of the talking. I eventually asked him if he would be willing to give me a ride to my car once we reached the top. Without hesitation he said yes. Part of me hoped he wasn't a serial killer, and the other part didn't care. My car was parked three miles away from the trailhead.

After rounding each switchback I was sure I would see the top but instead there was just another switchback. I finally told myself to stop wishing for that and instead put my energy into increasing my pace. My newfound partner was starting to fall behind and was forced to occasionally run to catch up with me. Each step, as uncomfortable as it was, felt like a micro victory. I only concentrated on the next step and then the step after that. I knew I was making good time because now Tim had stopped talking all together. Every time I looked over at him, he was gasping for air. The next time I looked forward, I saw the top and started to run. In between gasps Tim blurted out, "You're crazy!" as I reached the top but still kept moving. Tim finally caught up, giving me a giant high five and appeared to be as happy as I was. We continued walking to his car that was about 200 yards away. I hesitantly got into the passenger seat because I knew what was coming next. As soon as I closed the door both my calves and hamstrings seized and it made my eyes water. Tim asked if I was ok as I rocked back and forth in the seat. I was still wearing a smile and told him I had felt worse, which wasn't a lie. Rather than making him go out of his way, I had him drop me off in a parking lot that was adjacent to where my car was parked. I repeated the same words that were spoken to me a short time ago, telling Tim he was a good man while shaking his hand.

As I slowly shuffled to my car, I recorded this final message ...

"I'm back to where this all started in 12 hours and 23 minutes for the Rim to Rim to Rim. I found this cool dude who I came back the last mile with and gave me a ride to my car because it would have been a three mile walk. Epic, epic adventure! This last message I want to leave is called victim face. It's that self-defeated, feeling-sorry-for-yourself look. There's no place for that. When you get done with something and accomplish a great goal,

stand up tall. No lying on the ground. No hands on your knees. No sitting down. Put your chin up, chest out, and act like you are going to do it again because there may come a time when you have to. It's been awesome and I'll be talking to you soon."

I texted Bob to let him know I had finished, and this was our exchange-

Bob: Food and sleep. You have conquered the canyon.
Me: I think it was a tie.
Bob: Tying God is not such a bad thing.
Me: I felt Him.
Bob: Amen.

Although I finished 23 minutes past my time goal, I was still happy and proud of what I had accomplished. It wasn't because most people take a full day to complete this. It was because I knew how far I had personally come in my pursuit of personal greatness. I kept reminding myself of this as I struggled mightily to ascend a flight of stairs to my hotel room.

Chapter 14- The Grudge Match

After my 2018 Mind the Ducks race, I felt vindicated and relieved until the next time I drove by the course. It was my time to celebrate or at least that's what I thought. Instead of contrition, I got the cold stare of defiance from the course. It took me a few minutes to process it but then it hit me like a sledgehammer...we were tied. There was no clear victor, we were 1-1. I knew I needed to return and hopefully end this madness once and for all. The Grudge Match was born.

In 2019, I ran a different race that was for the position of Sheriff in Orleans County. The campaigning process took every minute of my spare time. It was more exhausting than ultra-training and left zero time for serious running. I lost the primary election by about 100 votes with over 3600 cast. It was a tough loss and I learned much from the experience. More importantly, I met many great people that I now call friends.

The following year the race was canceled due to the COVID 19 pandemic. In 2021 the race was originally canceled again but then moved to the fall. I already had a Colorado elk hunt planned for that timeframe. That hunt had me living in a tent in the high mountains by myself for nine days. It was a great adventure although no elk were harmed.

I was elated to learn the 2022 race was to be held on May 7th and began my official run training at the first of the year. I again did a weekly long run followed by next day backup runs. Half of these runs were done with my girlfriend Laura outside. The other half were completed on a noisy $125 garage sale treadmill in my basement with Pandora 80's rock playing in the background. These were spent studying and dissecting the man in the mirror while ramping up the speed every half mile or mile, depending on the length of the run, for hours on end. More negative split training. The man in the mirror would get a simple head nod of approval when the task was finished. I find no purpose in celebrating what absolutely needs to be done. On the rare occasions I tripped the breaker on the treadmill, he would get a, "Yeah, you did!" The two times he fell short, he was called, "A little punk ass bitch." Two other runs were completed each week, a faster tempo run and 1/4 mile repeats. These were also done utilizing negative splits.

During all of my training runs I tried to solely focus on the race and ran that mile loop hundreds of times in my head. I ran the first two hours of the race – calculated and reserved with zero concern about those ahead of me. This race wasn't about them however, I knew I would eventually paint targets on the backs of those in front of me. I ran hours three through eleven, confident and emotionless as possible, until the emotions boil over. They always boil over. I rarely get to choose which side of the coin I get- joy/sorrow, courage/fear, hope/despair. When the "good" emotions arise, I don't increase my pace but rather slow down my mind so I can stay in the moment. When the "bad" ones come, I always run faster. Demons rarely stick around if you punch them in the gut a few times. I have run the last hour- if my internal governor is still on, it gets turned off. The race morphs into no holds barred over that last hour.

I trained during those four months as if my life depended on it. I had retired in May of 2020, and no longer had work interfering with training. I didn't miss one session and continued the process of trying to break myself during each one. The goal was to match my mileage in 2018. I had the training completed, the goal set, and now I just needed to execute the plan.

Before I knew it, race day had arrived and I woke up well before the 4 am alarm sounded on my phone. I packed everything in my car the night before and just needed to eat and get dressed. I retrieved my "Team Pierson" shirt and slipped it over my head. It had been almost two years since I wore that tattered piece of armor. Every hair on my body stood on end and I was immediately reminded of a fallen hero and the men I call brothers. I was leaving nothing to chance today, and that shirt had protected me on more high-risk search warrants than I can count. It is one of my symbols of remembrance, duty, and honor.

I arrived at the race site an hour early and set up a small table to place my food and drink on. All of my supplies were packed in a sneaker box, and I also brought a metal folding chair in case I needed to sit and pop blisters during the race. I would have no crew today until Laura got out of work and had no pacers lined up. It was just me against the course and I felt its presence the moment I got out of my car. I knew it wanted to break me like it did in 2017. My job was not to break. I felt myself becoming anxious and relieved it by having this internal dialogue with the course while sitting on that cold chair. *I hope you weren't banking on that guy from 2017 showing up today. I burned him to the ground. He no longer exists, and you will never break me again. Get Father Time and round up all the demons you can find, but it still won't matter. It all ends today.*

At 7 am the race started, and I was among 175 other runners. Twelve of them bolted out in front of me and I stuck with the game plan of not caring what they did. Coincidentally the first song to play on my outdated iPod Nano was one that reminds me of certain people who have left this earth and now prosper in another realm. They include my mother, father, Fran McKenna, Daryl Pierson, Billy Mahoney, and Tom Valentine. I internally spoke the following to them, *I have never asked any of you for help during these trivial matters and today is no exception. I just hope I can get to a place of suffering where you feel I'm worthy of a visit.*

I settled into a comfortable pace and would quickly stop by my table after every 3 miles to grab a bottle of sports drink or water and some food. I would take them with me and eat and drink while running the next mile. My goal was to have very little downtime because every second mattered. My GPS watch would vibrate after each mile and display the time it took to complete it. I tried hard to keep each mile within 10 seconds of the one before it. I also tried to keep my emotions bottled up because it was much too early in the race for them to escape. At the four-hour mark, I had averaged a 9:36 minute mile pace and completed 25 miles which was exactly where I wanted to be.

I continued running proud and strong but dialed back the pace by about a minute per mile. This was also the plan and by now no one had passed me for several hours. I patiently waited for the halfway point to come because that was when the wheels came off in 2017. I let out a small laugh when it eventually arrived and muttered the word, "Nothing." Nothing hurt, no signs of weakness and zero negative thoughts. *I told you that guy was gone.*

While I had added a relatively small amount of time to my pace, I noticed most of the field had dramatically slowed and were showing signs of weariness. Many racers start out running a 12-hour race as if it was a 6-hour race. I had learned long ago that ultras don't really start until the second half. I ran the second four hours of the race averaging a 10:31 minute mile pace and started to feel fatigue setting in. You couldn't tell because I mostly maintained an expressionless look on my face, while also reminding myself to smile now and then. After all, this was completely voluntary. I soon began to sense my emotions starting to boil over. A blister had formed on the left ball of my foot and four of my toenails began to sting, a sure sign they were dying.

That's it? I asked the demons knowing full well they had more in store for me.

Laura arrived and the sight of her made me happy. She would prepare my drinks and food thus cutting down my refueling time. That doesn't mean I was in a good place though. Fatigue kept creeping into my body and the top of my right foot was becoming borderline painful. I have had issues with it since 2020 and the inflammation would come and go. *You knew this was going to happen! Deal with it like you dealt with it on your long runs.* I told myself. I continued trying to keep my right foot in the discomfort silo. Laura also ran numerous laps with me which helped to keep the demons at bay.

As I pressed on, my thoughts turned to my good friend Tom Drennan. I have known him for many years and it's hard to find a better man. A little over a year ago he was diagnosed with an aggressive form of blood cancer called multiple myeloma. This required him to undergo chemotherapy sessions, then stem cell replacement. Since the cancer is not curable, Tom requires monthly chemo "maintenance" treatments for the rest of his life. I would periodically call to check on his progress and not once did he feel sorry for himself. He always maintained a positive attitude and talked about "kicking cancer's ass."

I reminded myself that what I was doing pales in comparison to the suffering he endured during his treatments to get better. Slowly this was turning into the "Tom Drennan Race," and I couldn't be happier for I was honoring his indomitable spirit while also pummeling the course.

I could slowly feel the "shuffle" starting to happen which means my stride was beginning to shorten because of tired legs. Time began slowing down as each mile loop seemed to go on forever. It always fascinates me how easy an 11:00 minute pace feels on fresh legs but then resembles a sprint on fatigued lactic acid filled legs. The demons were still active in my blistered and sore feet and were also trying to influence my soul. They would say it was ok to walk because most of the other racers were, and no one would care. *I fucking care,* was my response as I fought hard to keep them at arm's length. The upside was the course no longer felt monotonous, so I began to loop one song on my iPod, Dierks Bentley's, *Burning Man*. It perfectly describes me as being the person I am now compared to the person I was, but that I am still far from righteous. It also reminds me of Badwater 135 when I thought the Joshua trees were coming to life and trying to attack me.

As I completed a lap around the nine hour mark, I saw Jay Vislay standing with Laura. He started running with me and it was like an instant shot of adrenaline. We ran lap after lap, and I was happy when he told me he was going to stay until the end of the race. What made me even happier was my SWAT brother Mat

Potocki and my son Zachary unexpectedly showed up. It is always a huge boost for me when I see loved ones on the course.

After what seemed much longer than 11 hours the final hour was upon me. My iPod battery had died, and this allowed me to solely concentrate on the rage I was feeling toward the course for making me feel so uncomfortable. My calves and quadriceps were on the verge of seizing and almost every part of my body was in distress. I railed against it by running faster while also realizing many bad things can happen in an hour. I methodically increased my pace while taunting the course with, *"That's all you got?"* I asked Laura how much time I had left in the race as I passed her. She told me 25 minutes and I started formulating my plan for finishing. A racer only gets credit for completed laps and I wanted to make every minute count. After calculating the pace for three more laps, I knew this would be far too aggressive considering my last lap had been 11 minutes and 26 seconds. I would have to settle on two more instead.

I fought hard on the next lap while reminding myself of the torment I felt after quitting the race in 2017. It took every ounce of energy to reverse the tired leg shuffle I had been doing over the last several hours. I passed racer after racer, who were mostly walking, and gave each of them a hearty, "Good job!" As I approached the end of that mile the demons chirped, "You don't need to push this hard, you have plenty of time." A small part of me agreed until I thought, *Why would you ruin this race by not finishing strong?* Just before completing that mile, Mat handed me a SWAT flag he had jerry-rigged to an axe handle. I would proudly fly those colors on my last lap. I told Jay I wanted to complete the final mile by myself because I needed one last solo duel with the course.

As I continued to run on, I heard a lady say, "I'm not sure he'll be able to make another lap." Before my internal governor that controls my mouth could catch it, a very sincere, "Fucking watch," came out of it. I pushed on but felt myself fading. *Come on, hang on,* I thought as I neared the 3/4 mile mark. Almost every Friday I do quarter mile repeats to help with my running speed. After warming up, I sprint a quarter mile followed by a slow paced "recovery" quarter mile. I repeat this process three to five times and try to make each sprint faster than the last. I do this by erasing my internal whiteboard of the physical and mental fatigue from the last sprint. In other words, I try to start fresh on each one. I knew I needed to do that now and it would take a pretty big eraser.

Stand by. Ready! Go! I told myself as my legs began to turn over. I felt myself gaining momentum and in that instant I saw her, my mother. She had her heartfelt loving smile that always made me feel loved. Before I could tell her I loved her, she was gone. I felt my eyes welling up with tears, but they weren't based in sorrow. Although I wished she would have stayed longer, I was so happy to see her because the last time was in 2016 at Badwater 135. Hyperventilation snapped me back to the task at hand although I desperately wanted to stay in that moment. I was in the middle of the giant flame and just had to hang on until the curve, at which point I would be able to see the finish line. I thought, *belly breathing, belly breathing.* It meant to breathe from the bottom of my lungs to combat my rapid-fire shallowing breathing. I desperately tried to find another gear as I reached the curve and headed for the finish. I crossed the line and continued running albeit at a slower pace. Even though I knew it didn't work that way, I wished my mother would return. I eventually stopped and was greeted with a congratulatory hug from Laura, Zachary, Jay, and Mat. It was finally over, and that last lap was my fastest of the race!

We made our way back to my aid station, but I refused to sit down. There was no way I would give the course that satisfaction. I couldn't really concentrate on what I had just accomplished because of numerous conversations with other racers that were passing by, while still hanging on to the thought of seeing my mother. When things started to quiet down, it sank in that I had ran 65.83 miles. I knew from a self-reflection standpoint that I had beat the course and this only confirmed it. I was both happy and relieved!

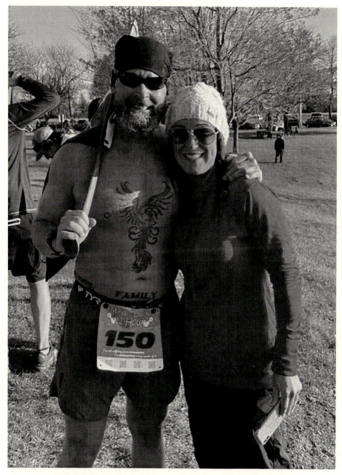

Celebrating with Laura after finishing the race

The crew helped me pack up my things and I told Laura I would be along shortly to her house which was nearby. After she left, I sat in my car while speaking to the course. "It was a great battle today and we both know who won. You can choose to accept it or don't, the choice is yours. Either way I am free of you." Even though my entire body was sore, I drove out of that parking lot with a peaceful soul. I had accomplished what I had set out to do. My only disappointment, which was mild at best, was I had given up a mile to Father Time. In 2018 I completed one additional mile. It served as a good reminder that he is always on the prowl. My efforts earned me first place again in the Male Veteran age group and fourth overall.

"What are you training for?" is a question I always get asked. I don't have a good answer for that right now. I am sure something will come along that interests me and manifests into a goal. This last race proved to me that I still have a lot left in the tank after entering the second half of my life. There is no true end game in mind other than living to the ripe old age of 100 while still remaining active. I do have a few adventures rattling around in my head and I am waiting for them to stick. The first one is running across the country. The trip would be approximately 2700 miles and take 103 days if I ran a 26.2 mile marathon every single day. Logistically, it would be a heavy lift because I would need someone to follow me in a car, or better yet a motorhome, the entire time. It would be a fantastic way to experience the various landscapes of our great country.

Another thought is trying to gain a birth in the famed Barkley Marathons. It's a five loop trail race which is roughly 100 miles in length with over 54,000 feet of accumulated vertical climb. There are time cutoffs for each loop, and one has to navigate during them to reach certain checkpoints. Most years no one finishes the race. Only 40 runners are chosen each year and receive a "letter of condolence" notifying them of their entry. It is considered by most to be the hardest trail race in the world.

My last idea is to become the oldest Ironman finisher in the world. The cutoff time to be considered an official finisher is 17 hours and there are also cutoff times for the 2.2 mile swim and 112 mile bike portions. Currently there is a gentleman who completed the race at 85 years of age in 2018 and plans on competing into his 90's. Optimistically, I have over 30 years to get over my disdain for bike riding and train for it. It would be a great adventure at that age!

Chapter 15- Revelations from a Gray Man

Mental toughness reigns supreme in whatever you do in life.

On May 25th, 2020, I retired after 32 years of service in law enforcement. I was looking for a way to celebrate my retirement but there were no races due to COVID. I remembered something SWAT brother Mat Potocki told me about a book he had read. It was written by a Navy SEAL. The author said if you really want to find out about yourself, strap on a backpack and walk for 24 hours.

I first met Mat when he was in the academy. He spoke very little and his form during physical training sessions was perfect. Even after especially hard training evolutions, he would always stand straight up with a stoic look on his face. Later, Mat made the SWAT Team and was eventually assigned to my squad. He quickly became one of my go-to guys. Mat would arrive an hour early to everything and volunteer for even the shittiest assignments. I decided I was going to run/walk for 24 hours for my retirement celebration and asked Mat to join me since he put the idea in my head. Thanks Mat! Without an ounce of hesitation, he agreed to Wandering the Earth.

There are some things you should know about Mat. He absolutely despises running. Mat trains at Wolf

Brigade Gym under the tutelage of Greg Walsh. Greg is arguably one of the best strength and conditioning coaches in the word. He is also Mat's mentor. Greg's process produces extraordinary individuals and some of his tenets are perfect form, mental toughness, and a sense of community. One of his principles I now live by, is after even extremely difficult physical challenges, stand up straight and look and act like you have to do it again. No flopping on the ground or defeated hands-on knees posture. When I think back to my bent-over, leaning-against-the-wall Louisville Ironman pose, I cringe a little, but also realize you don't know what you don't know. The only running Mat did to prepare was a few hill repeats near his house.

On June 6th at 8 am, we departed the police academy and began Wandering the Earth. We headed west and ran most of the first 50 miles. This was impressive because Mat had never run a total of 50 miles during his lifetime. He optimistically exclaimed we should be well over our goal of 100 miles at 24 hours. I lied and agreed knowing things would eventually slow down. They did but Mat soldiered on without complaint. I could tell by his gait that his feet and ankles were hurting, but I saw not one ounce of suffering in his face. We completed 85 miles and I sensed Mat was hiding his disappointment of not reaching 100 miles. For me, it was great spending 24 hours with a brother I had so much respect and admiration for.

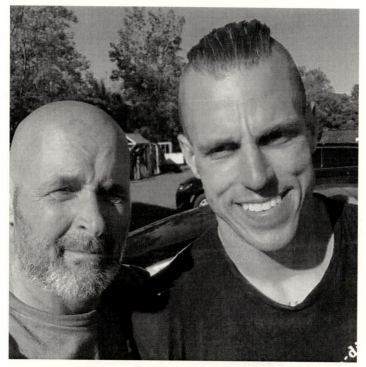

Brother Mat after Wandering the Earth- Part I

In late September, the call that I knew was inevitable had finally come. Mat wanted to try it again and make 100 miles this time. To be completely honest, it was probably the last thing I wanted to do because my ankle was still healing from my Grand Canyon run, but I would never tell Mat no to anything. This time my house would serve as home base, so we didn't have to waste time going into stores to resupply food and drink. I set up a tent at the end of my driveway to house everything we needed. On October 3rd we began Wandering the Earth- Part II although I wasn't quite sure Mat had fully recovered from the first one. He did absolutely zero running in preparation for this one. We ran mile after mile with almost no walking. Mat once again remained stoic the entire time and completed the 100 miles in 22 hours and 33 minutes. He went 15 miles further in 1 ½ hours of less time compared to the initial one. Mat was not born with mental toughness and grit. They were forged through adversity, self-discipline, and good old fashioned hard work. We should all be more like Mat.

We currently live in an instant gratification society. True change takes time and does not happen overnight. Lasting change occurs in small stages, and this helps to make your foundation sturdy. Whether it is losing weight, gaining weight, getting stronger or developing better aerobic capacity, it is more likely to stick if these gains are built incrementally and without shortcuts. Fads come and go while hard work and perseverance endures the test of time. My journey started in 2001, and over twenty years later I am still evolving for the better. I often think back to that dreadful 5K in which my sons beat me and I'm glad I didn't give up. The key component is that you must wholeheartedly desire the change. It can't be dictated by someone else. You need your own meaningful buy in.

Motivation has turned into a somewhat of a bad word nowadays. I think it can be beneficial when you are first starting out in your training or transformation.

Motivation will initially get you out of bed when you are tired however, it will eventually wane. The key is to use motivation to develop self-discipline which can be long lasting. Self-discipline aids in removing your "feelings" from the equation. You do what needs to be done despite not wanting to do it. Excuse my crude saying, "Fuck your feelings." Feelings often get in the way and muddy the waters when it comes to completing very meaningful training. I rarely "feel" great before every session, but it still needs to be completed with a high amount of effort.

A written plan can be essential for staying on course. You wouldn't build a house without a blueprint and a plan is just that. Following a well thought out plan helps to develop self-discipline and ensures you do what is required. It also reinforces the sense of accomplishment. I look at it as a 'Honey Do" list. It's a very satisfying experience to systematically cross off a list of chores over the course of a week. This is the same thing. I always print off my training schedule, then highlight the sessions after their completion. This also serves as a red flag should I notice a lack of highlights over the course of a week or month. Make no mistake, self-discipline is perishable.

Surround yourself with family and friends who are supportive of you -- people that are positive and make you a better person. There will be some who won't understand your journey and that's fine. Accept help and advice from those who do because your success will likely become their success. Dismiss the naysayers and use their negativity as fuel. The most important thing is to do you. Find your own personal greatness. It's okay to have idols and role models but never compare yourself to them. If you must do a comparison, let it be of where you are now in relation to where you started.

It's perfectly fine to have a "down season" to re-charge your batteries and reset. It's rarely ok to not do anything, but better to dial it back and regroup. You just need to know the difference between dreading a workout because it's going to be difficult and dreading a workout because you are burned out. The key is to have longevity rather than being a flash in the pan.

The term "diet" is something most people are concerned with and the name itself conjures up many different thoughts, most of them being negative. The most prominent are the various fads you are constantly bombarded with. There are the Atkins, Paleo, Vegetar-ian, Vegan, Intermittent Fasting and the like. I believe the best "diet" is the one that is realistic and sustainable for you and your lifestyle. I am not a proponent of the current food pyramid and believe protein should make up the bulk of your intake followed by vegetables and fruit. It is unrealistic to completely eliminate carbohy-drates such as pasta, grains, and bread, but they should probably be the smallest thing on your plate. It's okay to cheat here and there and indulge in food you ordinarily don't eat. The fundamental thing to remember is mod-eration is key.

It took me many years to differentiate between pain and discomfort and this is still a work in progress. Early on, I often mistook discomfort for pain. For me, pain is burning my hand on a hot stove or breaking my toe on a piece of furniture. It causes me to want to hold the affected area. Discomfort on the other hand is bothersome but bearable such as a cramp in my side when running or a blister forming on my heel. There are various levels of both and it's important not to intermingle the two. You can train to bear and even embrace discomfort during your quest for personal greatness. The more you can take, the greater you can become. Constant and consistent exposure to discomfort also allows you to start placing things you initially thought to be painful into the discomfort silo. Once you begin doing that, new doors will open for you both physically and more importantly mentally. It's a proven fact our minds give up well before our bodies are ready to do so.

You will get sore or injured if you immerse yourself in meaningful training. The key is to mitigate it and recover as quickly as possible. I use the acronym **R.I.I.M. R** is for rest. I don't stop training all together if my patellar tendon becomes inflamed. I will do other activities such as swimming, elliptical and cycling that don't aggravate the area. **I** is for ice, which is a miracle drug. I often take ice baths after long runs or when I feel inflammation starting to set in. When there wasn't time for one, I would tape sandwich bags filled with ice to my knees for the 30 minute drive to work. The second **I** is

Ibuprofen. If you have lingering bouts of inflammation, your best course of action may be prescription strength doses of NSAID's. I would take 800 mgs (four over the counter 200mg tablets) three times a day with food for a week. The area will start feeling better after the first day but that does not mean the inflammation is gone. You need a steady stream of it in your body for it to be effective against the root cause of the inflammation. **M** is for massage. Depending on the area, I use an electric hand-held massager, foam roller, beaded stick roller, lacrosse ball and a massage chair I bought as a retirement gift for myself. Most of these aid in releasing the lactic acid in my muscles. I follow up by consuming steady amounts of water to purge the free-floating lactic acid through urination. I know I am on the right track when the toilet bowl is full of foam after I urinate.

Be happy for other people's successes. We have turned into a society where many are trying to keep up with the Joneses. That would all end if we just kept up with ourselves. It means having your own unique aspirations and setting your own goals. Make your life great and rejoice when others do the same thing. Being kind to others is free. While fishing in Canada as a young man with my father, I met Mike Knott. He was a man who was always upbeat and positive. I visited him one weekend and as we walked to a diner for breakfast, he had a sincere greeting for everyone that passed -- "Hello," "Good morning" and the like. The curiosity finally got to me, and I asked if he knew all those people. He replied no and asked why. I told him I wasn't sure why he addressed everyone if they were complete strangers. His retort has stuck with me for the past 35 years. That a kind word doesn't cost you a cent and might be the nicest thing that person hears all day. Those are some of the truest words ever spoken to me.

My sincere hope is that you experience personal greatness. Know that your shade of gray does not limit true personal greatness. Allow yourself to get in over your head because that is where you will evolve the most. Set out to obtain a lofty goal and train for it like your life depends on it. This may very well be the case depending on the goal. I guarantee your perspective on life will change once you obtain it.

About the Author

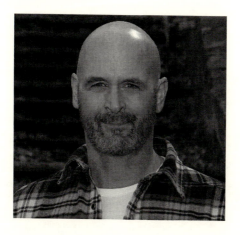

Brett Sobieraski refers to himself as a gray man — an average man that travels mostly unnoticed throughout life. Despite having self-proclaimed subpar athletic abilities, he has completed Badwater 135, numerous 100-mile ultra-marathons, double Ironman, swam 32 miles across Lake Ontario and ran for 50 hours to benefit Special Olympics. He often raises money for charities during his races.

Happily retired after being a police officer for 32 years, Brett worked mostly in narcotics and was also on the SWAT Team at the Rochester Police Department. Additionally, Brett was an instructor at the police academy who taught physical fitness and narcotics training until his retirement. Brett loved shaping new officers' minds and bodies. Brett feels he left his job with his sanity, a positive outlook, and a strong sense of humanity.

Brett is proof that personal greatness can be achieved by anyone if they are willing to make substantial sacrifices. He enjoys mentoring and supporting others in their quests. Brett learned that training his mind was more important than training his body, discovering that mental toughness is the cornerstone to his successes. His feats have been the result of incremental changes to his lifestyle, coupled with a knack for getting in over his head, like the time he built his own house.

To learn more about and to connect with Brett on social media, visit his website, www.graymaninc.com

Made in United States
North Haven, CT
11 June 2023

37623456R00129